SPECTACULAR
SEX MOVES
HE'LL NEVER FORGET

INGENIOUS POSITIONS AND TECHNIQUES THAT WILL BLOW HIS MIND

Text © 2010 Sonia Borg, Ph.D., MA, M.P.H.
Photography © 2010 Quiver

First published in the USA in 2010 by
Quiver, a member of
Quayside Publishing Group
100 Cummings Center
Suite 406-L
Beverly, MA 01915-6101
www.quiverbooks.com

The Publisher maintains the records relating to images in this book required by
18 USC 2257. Records are located at Rockport Publishers, Inc., 100 Cummings Center,
Suite 406-L, Beverly, MA 01915-6101.

A Note to Readers:
This book contains the opinions and ideas of the author and is intended for the
use of informed and consenting adults. It's not therapy; it's fun.

Sonia Borg, Ph.D., MA, M.P.H. is a clinical sexologist, not a therapist or medical doctor.
Some of the practices and positions in this book may not be appropriate for people
with medical conditions or physical impairments. Use your good judgment!

ISBN-13: 978-1-59233-425-4
ISBN-10: 1-59233-425-3

Library of Congress Cataloging-in-Publication Data
Borg, Sonia.
   Spectacular sex moves he'll never forget : ingenious positions and techniques
   that will blow his mind / Sonia Borg.
       p.   cm.
   Includes bibliographical references and index.
   ISBN-13: 978-1-59233-425-4 (alk. paper)
   ISBN-10: 1-59233-425-3 (alk. paper)
   1. Sex instruction for women. 2. Sexual intercourse. 3. Male orgasm. I. Title.
      HQ46.B674 2010
      613.9'6--dc22

                                                        2010028622

Book design by Holtz Design
Photography by Holly Randall
Illustrations by Robert Brandt
Printed and bound in Singapore

SONIA BORG PH.D., M.A., M.P.H.
AUTHOR OF *ORAL SEX HE'LL NEVER FORGET*

SPECTACULAR SEX MOVES HE'LL NEVER FORGET

INGENIOUS POSITIONS <u>AND</u> TECHNIQUES THAT WILL BLOW <u>HIS</u> MIND

QUIVER

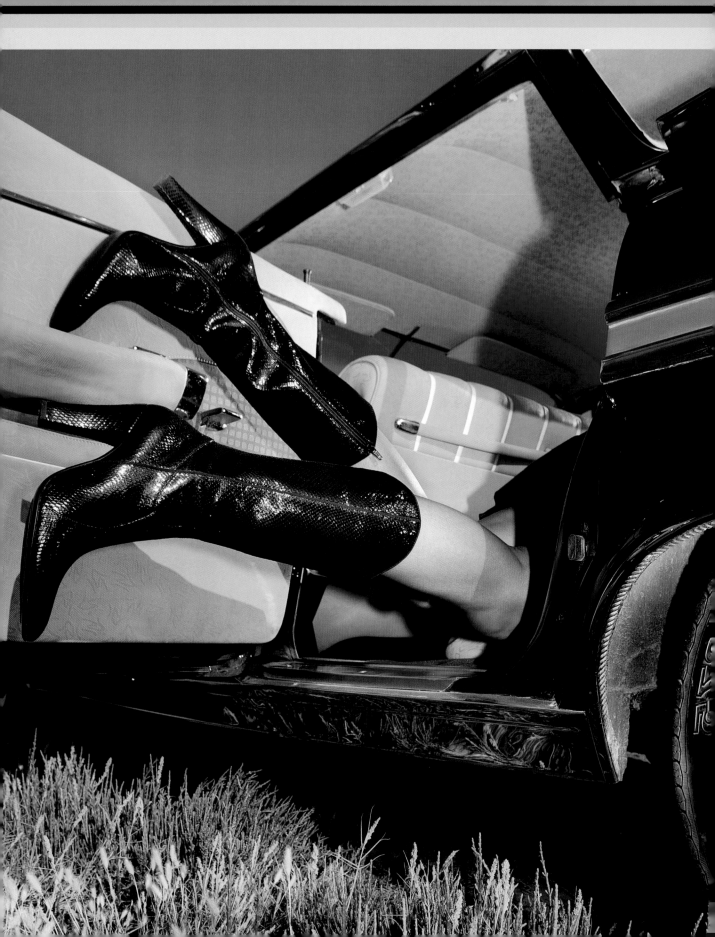

Contents

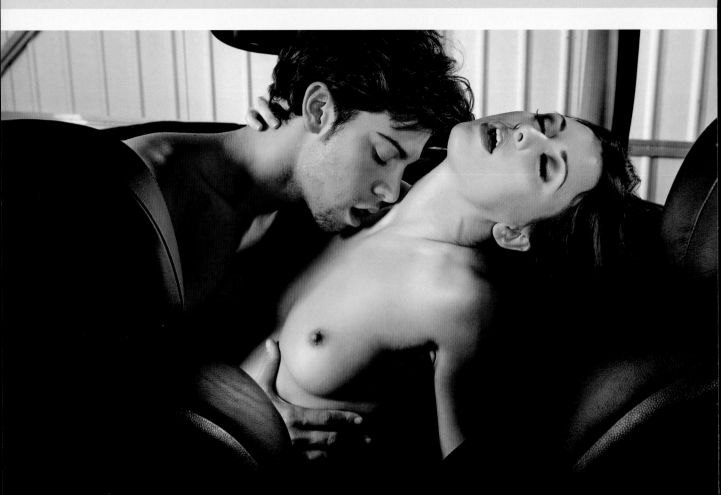

 # INTRODUCTION

So, what does a man want in bed? Well, according to research, the best predictors of sexual satisfaction for men is changing sexual positions.

And so this book was born. *Spectacular Sex Moves He'll Never Forget* was created out of the need for men and women to better satisfy each other sexually. Generally, men communicate better physically and women verbally. Instead of waiting for the day that he becomes better at communicating verbally, try entering his world, the world of the physical.

This book will teach you how to move and navigate with a man to total and complete sexual satisfaction (his and yours) through sexual positioning. In the process you will discover:

★ Increased confidence in your own skill-set as a lover

★ A new form of communication that will energize and empower you

★ A newly inspired sense of sexual adventure and creativity

★ A sense of freedom from living outside your comfort zone, having sex, and living life differently

★ And I promise this to both you and your lover: The relationship will feel new and exciting again.

The book is organized into different sections so you can master positioning quickly and easily: He's on Top, Rear Entry, She's on Top, Sitting, Standing, Side by Side, Blow Job Positions, Hand Jobs, and More Happy Endings.

Although other books may teach you different position techniques as I do here, my book does more than that! I have created special scenarios that turn sex into an event. Each scenario is exciting and creative and will help you master positioning.   There is a scenario for every erotic mood. In addition, Sex Facts are sprinkled throughout the book and are sure to add to your sexual knowledge. Within the scenarios, you'll find easy segments:

★ Preparations gives you all the little preparatory details,

★ Lead In guides you through the first step and helps initiate the act,

★ Foreplay lays down a unique and appropriate warm up to . . .

★ The Main Act, which gives you step-by-step directions from first touch to orgasm. You will always know what to do next.

★ Why it Works for Her and Why it Works for Him will explain the "why" behind the move, multiplying your sexual knowledge and increasing your sexual satisfaction.

★ And finally, The Sexpert Says, gives you useful information based on my own experience, observations as a clinical sexologist, and confessions from clients. The notes here will help you understand how to be creative, light, and playful with sex. It will give you a snapshot of male sexuality with some insights into female sexuality, too.

There is a positions scenario here for every mood, from playful to soul-mate connecting . If you try one and don't like it, try another… and another…. and another. Adapt, change, and modify to make each your own.

I sincerely hope that my book will give you the tools and inspiration for rocking his erotic world.

Wishing you a healthy and happy sex life!
xoxox,

Dr. Sonia

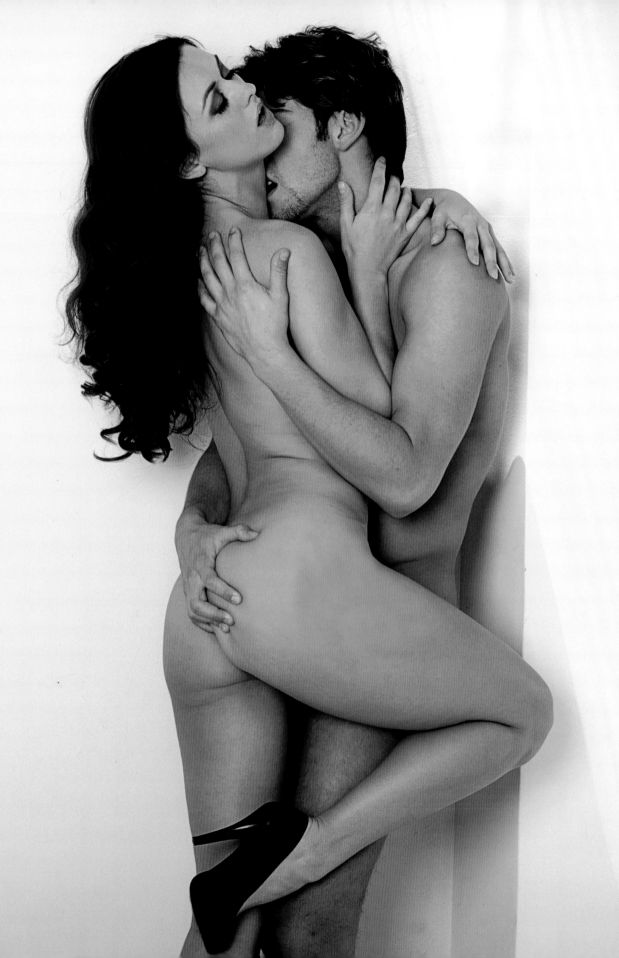

But First, Basic Male Anatomy: You've Got to Know His Parts

Although you have an up-close and personal relationship with his penis and testicles, you may not know how each part functions to create that dynamic male sex organ. Before we get into blow jobs, here's a quick tutorial on his private and prized parts.

THE TESTICLES AND THEIR PACKAGE

Think of this area as his little production company. Like your ovaries, it produces the material necessary for propagating the species—in his case, sperm. While your sex hormones are also produced in smaller quantities in the uterus, his sex hormone, testosterone, comes entirely from this part of his body. This package contains:

★ **The Testicles: Testes or Gonads (in common vernacular: "Balls")** Held together by the baggy skin of the scrotum, his testicles are located behind his penis. They not only produce testosterone and sperm, but they also store it. When he gets excited, his balls rise closer to his penis, making the path to ejaculation more efficient.

★ **The Scrotum (also known as "the Sack")**
The scrotum is the soft, delicate, baggy sack of skin protecting his testicles. Its primary function is maintaining body temperature conducive to the survival of sperm. Ever wonder why his balls shrink up in the cold? The skin of the scrotum tightens, pulling the testicles up closer to his body for the heat.

THE PENIS OR PHALLUS (KNOWN AS DICK, COCK, PRICK, THROBBING MANHOOD, AND SO FORTH)

His penis has two biological functions: channeling urine out of the body and ejaculating sperm-containing semen. Composed of secondary fibrous connective tissue and smooth muscles, the penis is mainly spongy (erectile) tissue laced with veins and arteries that fill with blood when he is aroused. Its skin covering is thin and silky to the touch.

SEX FACT

The size of flaccid penises varies more widely than that of erect penises. A small penis actually grows more with erection than a large one does, making erections more equal than men realize.

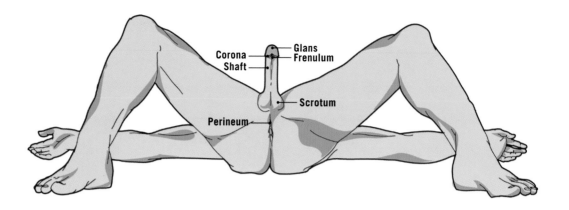

The sections of the penis are:

★ **The Shaft (or Rod)** The main body of his organ, the shaft connects the head and the scrotum. This is the power part of the penis—the area that becomes engorged with blood during arousal. As you already know, it is capable of amazing growth when properly inspired. **The Head (or Glands)** The big, beautiful head rides proudly atop the shaft, where it resembles a helmet. The most sensitive part of the penis, the head is porous and secretes small beads of lubrication, sometimes called pre-cum. (Yes, it can contain sperm.)

★ **Foreskin (or Prepuce)** Many of you may never have seen an adult male with foreskin, the loose skin covering the head of the penis. In modern Western (and some other) societies, the skin is removed at birth or shortly after in the procedure known as circumcision. An uncircumcised penis appears to be wearing a turtleneck sweater. The head is not visible when the penis is flaccid.

★ **Frenulum** The piece of tissue connecting the head of the penis to the shaft is called the frenulum. The connecting line looks like a V on the underside of the penis. Often neglected in fellatio, the frenulum is very sensitive. Don't overlook it!

★ **Corona (or Ridge)** The aptly named corona is that ridge of flesh where the head of the penis rises above the shaft. It looks like a crown, hence the name *corona*. You probably give it a lot of attention when you suck the head. Irresistible, isn't it?

THE FORGOTTEN ZONE

You may be squeamish about going there. Or he may be the one who shies away from contact below the balls. But this is rich sexual territory. It includes:

★ **Anus (or Butthole)** The anus, his and yours, has a high concentration of nerve endings. Stimulation is pleasurable unless the receiver is not prepared for touch or adamantly rejects the idea. If he's willing, use a well-greased finger or two, protected by disposable finger cots (little plastic gloves for your fingertips), and proceed with care.

★ **Perineum (also known as the Taint, as in "It t'aint your balls and it t'aint your ass")** The space between his anus and the base of his scrotum is the perineum. It doesn't have the same negative connotations for most men that the anus may have. Press your thumb or finger pad lightly into the area and see how he responds. You can bring some guys to orgasm by pressing that magic button.

★ **Prostate (or Male G-Spot)** You can't see his G-spot; it's hidden inside, like yours is. Located between the rectum and the bladder, the prostate is behind the perineum. It may be more effectively stimulated by anal play. If applying pressure to his perineum doesn't seem to do anything for him, coax him into letting you put a finger inside his anus. Stroke in the direction of his prostate.

PUBOCOCCYGEUS (PC) MUSCLE

You and your man have more than G-spots in common. Every woman surely knows about her PC muscle by now. Yet few men do. His PC muscle, like yours, controls urine flow and contracts during orgasm. If he exercises that muscle, it will become stronger, enhancing his sexual performance and intensifying his orgasm. He should be doing the male version of Kegel exercises (see "How to Find Your (and His) PC Muscle" later in this section for more information). If he has a well-toned PC muscle, he will be able to move his erect penis up and down.

But First, Basic Female Anatomy: You've Got to Know Your Own Parts

You can't expect to drive him crazy unless you know how to drive your own car. Here is a breakdown of your parts.

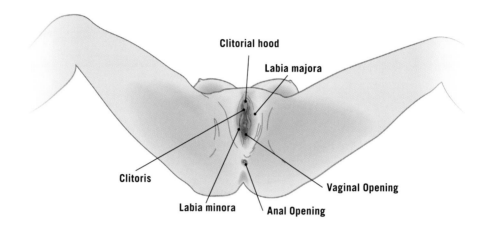

THE VULVA (AKA PUSSY, YONI)

The vulva, by its politically and anatomically correct name, is the whole package of the female genitalia:

★ **Mons or Mons Veneris (Latin for *Mound of Venus*)** This soft spot on top of the pubic bone is sensitive to the touch and nice for arousal, but stimulation there generally won't take you to climax.

★ **Labia Majora (Large Outer Lips)** The labia majora is a somewhat sensitive area that overlays and protects the more delicate inner layer of the vulva. The mons and outer lips are covered with hair (that some women wax or shave). Many women find that removing the hair increases sensitivity to touch.

★ **Labia Minora (Smaller Inner Lips)** These more sensitive lips swell and change color when you become aroused. They are more slender than the outer lips, though they sometimes extend past them.

THE CLITORIS (SLANG TERMS INCLUDE: THE LITTLE GIRL IN THE BOAT, THE BEAN, THE MAGIC BUTTON, THE PEARL, ETC.)

The clitoris is the only organ on the human body (male or the female) designed solely for pleasure.

The clitoris has 8,000 nerve endings and operates within a network of 15,000 nerve endings that service the entire pelvic region. Knowing this reminds you that it would be nearly impossible to have an orgasm that is not clitoral in nature.

Here are the components of the clitoris:

★ **The Clitoral Hood** This little outgrowth of skin covers and protects the clitoral glans. When a woman becomes aroused, the glans protrudes from the hood, though in some women, just barely.

★ **The Clitoral Glans or Shaft** When people refer to the clitoris, they usually mean the clitoral glans. The vast system of nerves connecting the clitoris to the vagina all end in the glans. What a potent little piece of genital property that is!

★ **The Crura (aka Wings)** *Crus* translates as "leg," thus *crura* means "legs." Located to the right and left of the urethra, the crura run back to the pubic bone. These two sections, the internal portion of the clitoris, are shaped like an inverted V, connecting to the clitoris at the point of that V.

★ **The Vestibular or Clitoral Bulbs** A string of bulb-shaped aggregations of erectile tissue, the clitoral bulbs extend down beneath the labia minora. When a woman is aroused, they fill with blood, making the vulva swell.

★ **The Fourchette** Technically translated, *fourchette* means "dessert fork." This refers to the bottom edges of the lips beneath the vaginal entrance, neighboring the perineum.

THE VAGINA

The vagina is the elastic, muscular canal connecting the uterus to the outside of the body. When you become aroused, the vagina expands in width and length and produces lubrication, though additional lube may be needed.

THE CERVIX

The narrow end of the uterus that connects it with the top of the vagina is the cervix. It feels hard to the touch and expands with arousal and orgasm. Some women report that stimulation to the anterior (anterior fornix erogenous zone, or AFE zone) and posterior fornices surrounding the cervix offers an intense orgasm and an emotional release. Other women report that the fornices can't be stimulated without contact to the cervix, which can be painful at times and arousing at others. The fornices have been described as a ringlike structure that encircles the cervix, with the texture similar to the back of a Frisbee.

G-SPOT

The much-hyped G-spot is a spongy, walnut-sized mass of tissue approximately 1 to 3 inches (2.5 to 7.5 cm) up on the back wall of the vagina. You can feel it by inserting two fingers into the vagina and making a "come hither" gesture.

Urine exits the body through the urethral opening. A small mass of erectile tissue above and on either side of that opening is very sensitive to erotic stimulation. Known as the U-spot, it is relatively undiscovered territory for some.

BARTHOLIN'S GLANDS

Located slightly below and to the left and right of the vaginal opening, Bartholin's glands secrete small quantities of lubrication when aroused.

SKENE'S GLANDS

Located behind the rear wall of the vagina and around the lower end of the urethra, Skene's glands swell with blood during arousal.

ANUS

The end of the colon, the anus is also very rich in nerve endings. Some women enjoy having their anus stimulated with a finger, a tongue, an anal dildo, or a penis. Both men and women have a sphincter muscle that controls opening and closing the anus and that also contracts at the point of orgasm.

PC MUSCLE

This is a hammocklike muscle stretching across the floor of the vagina from pubic bone to tailbone; it controls urine flow and contracts during orgasm. If you—both men and women—exercise that muscle, it will become stronger, enhancing sexual pleasure and intensifying orgasm for both of you. With a strong PC muscle, you will be able to grip his penis, and even pull it in and out of your vagina.

SEX FACT

Any place can be an erogenous zone. Sex researcher Alfred Kinsey found that some women could reach orgasm by having their earlobes nibbled or eyebrows stroked.

Doing Kegel exercises builds that muscle. For women, regular Kegels keep the vagina toned after childbirth and postmenopause. But Kegel exercises to strengthen the PC muscle are essential for every woman and man. Doing them is the absolute bottom-line requirement for good sex. Not only does a strong PC make your orgasm more likely and more intense, but it also facilitates multiple and extended orgasms. So do your Kegels!

How to Find Your (and His) PC Muscle

Locate your PC muscle by stopping and starting the flow of urine. Once you have located the muscle, begin with a short Kegel sequence.

Contract the muscle twenty times at approximately one squeeze per second. Exhale gently as you tighten only the muscles around your genitals (which includes the anus), not the muscles in your buttocks. Don't bear down when you release. Simply let go. Do two sets twice a day. Gradually build up to two sets of seventy-five per day.

Then add a long Kegel sequence. Hold the muscle contraction for a count of three. Relax between contractions. Work up to holding for ten seconds, then relaxing for ten seconds. Again, start with two sets of twenty each and build up to seventy-five.

Once you are doing 300 repetitions a day of the combined short and long sequences, you will be ready to add the push-out.

After relaxing the contraction, push down and out gently, as if you were having a bowel movement with your PC muscle. Repeat gently. No bearing down.

Now create Kegel sequences that combine long and short sets with push-outs. After a month of daily repetitions of 300, you should have a well-developed PC muscle. You can keep it that way simply by doing sets of 150 several times a week.

A VARIATION FOR HER: THE KEGEL CRUNCH

Vary your Kegel routine by doing them while exercising. For example, do Kegels as you perform pelvic crunches. Contract your PC as you pull in your stomach muscles. Release both at the same time.

A VARIATION FOR HIM: ADD WEIGHT

As his PC muscle grows stronger, he can perform exercises with first a damp handkerchief, then a face cloth, and finally a hand towel draped over his penis.

Penises and Their Types

All penises are unique and perfect for different reasons. Here are a few of the common types of penises and the different ways to play with them to get the most bang for your bucking pleasure.

LONGER

You can wrap both hands around his penis and have room to take him in your mouth, too. He can usually get your G-spot and your C-spot (cervix). Sometimes it hurts so good and other times it just hurts.

If this is you, try the following standing-up positions (described later in the book) that work well with the long schlong: Dressed to Thrill, Up Against the Wall, and Quiet Riot. The Stimulus Plan and Shoots and Ladders are excellent you-on-top, you-in-control positions that will allow you to get just the depth you need. You can also do Slinging Dixie, Dinner for Two, and Spring Fever when your legs are closed and his thighs are outside of yours, making the journey to your vagina longer and less direct.

SHORTER

With proper positioning, the shorter penis can be aimed so it directly hits the G-spot, which is just past the vaginal opening. Women with shorter vaginal canals, women who do not enjoy cervical stimulation, and women who love the thrill of deep throating him enjoy the shorter penis.

If you experience slip-outs, use less lube and wipe down natural lubrication with a towel. Flex your PC muscles and bear down a bit on the release to stimulate the head of his penis and other spots on you. Appreciate the magic of this penis type in the G-Works, the Hard Rock, and the intercourse variation of the Bouncing Ball Hand Job.

THINNER

Newbies to sex and women who have a tighter vagina report enjoying a thinner penis, which can go directly to all the spots without the distraction of feeling stretched. If you enjoy the friction of his penis against your vaginal walls, use less lube and wipe down natural lubrication with a towel. Practice strengthening your PC muscles. You could also narrow the vaginal canal from the inside by using beads or a butt plug inside your anus during sex.

LARGER CIRCUMFERENCE

Some women love the fullness, widening, and stretching feelings that a penis with thicker girth can provide. If you would like a smoother entrance, try using more lube. Have him enter you more slowly, or start with something smaller like a dildo or have him orally stimulate you so you can relax until you can graduate to taking in his penis.

CURVY

Curvy penises are fun to play with because you can use the curve to get that perfect G-spot stimulation. Squat or sit on the penis facing the direction it points and drop your pelvis down and back.

DEGREES OF HARDNESS

Penises may vary in degrees of hardness. Some penises do not ever get very hard. This could be due to diet or even age. Over time, plaque builds up in the arteries of the penis, just like in the heart, and inhibits the flow of blood to the penis. Other penises will be hard but their ligaments are stretched, causing them to become hard pointing in the downward position.

For softer penises, start off with one of the hand job or blow job positions. You could also try rear-entry positions like Head Over Wheels, with your butt lifted, or missionary with your legs up and around his back, where he's in control and can manage the slip-outs.

UNCIRCUMCISED

In many cultures, foreskin is removed from the penis (circumcision), whereas in other cultures, the skin is left on (uncircumcision). All of the positions listed in this book work great for both types of penis, but the uncircumcised man may feel additional sensations when you gently pull and hold down the skin at the base of the penis. There is a chapter titled "Exposed" in my book *Oral Sex He'll Never Forget* that goes into detail on how to give a great BJ to a man with an uncircumcised penis. But, basically, when giving a blow job, gently glide a lubed hand over the head and bring the loose skin down to the base, where you position your thumb and forefinger as if it were a cock ring.

SEX FACT

According to the *Glamour*/AOL.com sex survey, when asked "Which would you rather be: 5'2" tall with a 7-inch penis, or 6'2" tall with a 3-inch penis?" 68 percent would go for the larger penis. The same source also reports that 67 percent of men have measured their penis. The average penis size is 2 to 4 inches (5 to 10 centimeters) soft, 5 to 7 inches (13 to 18 centimeters) hard.

His Sexual Response Cycle

There are general stages of arousal common to all of us, yet specific to each of us. Paying attention to your lover's sexual response cycle (SRC) will make you the best lover he or she has ever had.

SIGNS OF EARLY AROUSAL

★ His heart rate increases and his blood pressure rises.

★ His body muscles tense.

★ His penis and nipples become engorged with blood and erect.

★ His testicles rise closer to his body.

APPROACHES

★ Psychologically and physically engage him.

★ Approach him with authentic appreciation.

★ Initiate physical contact with:

—Soft kisses

—Relaxed eye contact

—Light touches

—Long slow strokes and gradual builds are generally desirable at this initial stage.

AS HE BECOMES MORE AROUSED

★ His breathing deepens, and he may moan or gasp.

★ He sweats.

★ The corona becomes more prominent.

★ Drops of seminal fluid, or pre-cum, appear on the head of his penis.

APPROACHES

★ Incorporate a rhythm.

★ Establish patterns and sets.

★ Apply pressure.

★ Increase pace.

★ Apply direct contact to the head of the penis, balls, and other erogenous spots.

★ Try sucking, which works well to direct energy.

★ Create gaps or moments of no stimulation.

★ Be present, watching and listening to what he likes.

AS HE APPROACHES ORGASM

★ His heart rate, breathing, and blood pressure reach their peak.

★ His thrusting reaches a peak.

★ His body flushes.

★ He makes particular noises and may suddenly go stiff, signs that he has reached the point of ejaculatory inevitability. (You can't stop him now.)

APPROACHES

Continue whatever you did to get him to this point.

DURING ORGASM

★ He loses muscle control.

★ His penis contracts as he ejaculates.

★ The contractions may spread throughout his genitals, even into the rest of his body.

APPROACHES

As he winds down and his contractions become further apart, slow down the pace, lighten the pressure, and lessen the suction and direct stimulation to the head of the penis.

Depending on a number of factors, including age, the refractory period in men—the time before they can achieve another erection—may last anywhere from five minutes to twenty-four hours or more.

The better you know his genitals and his SRC, the more expertly you can play with his penis and get it to do what you want, when you want.

|||||||||||||||||||||||||||||||||||||||||||||||||||||||||||||||||||||||||||||||||||||||||||||||||||||||||||||||||||||||||||||||||||||||

THE SEXPERT SAYS

The best lovers are informed lovers. For more information, tips, and access to the author's video library, go to www.TheHappyEndingsCompany.com.

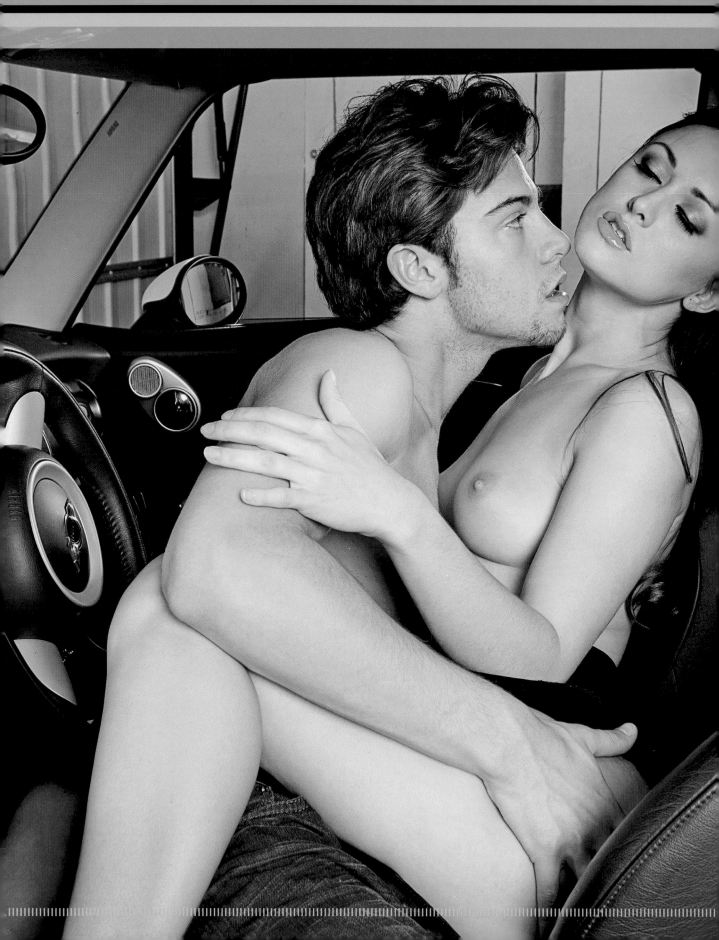

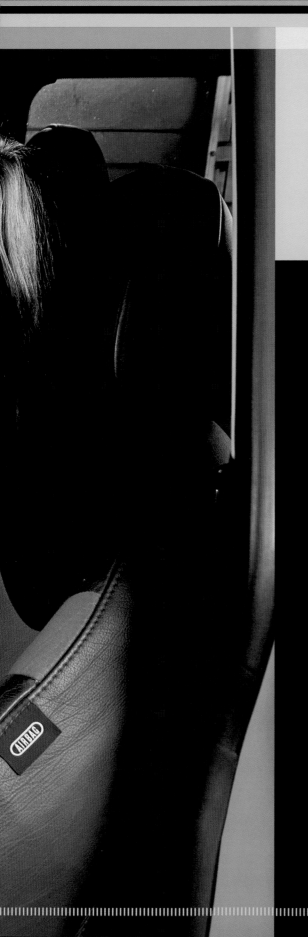

He's on Top

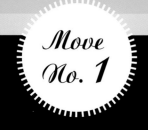

SLINGING DIXIE
(SEX IN A SEAT-BELT SLING)

If there is something men might love more than sex, it's their cars. There may even be times when you can't get between a man and his biggest toy. Don't try to fight it! Befriend the car. Together, you can create an experience that is sure to make his rod hot.

Since the automobile rolled onto the scene in the twentieth century, cars have been the no-cost motel on wheels for many lovers. Before you sigh and say "How boring!" or "What a cliché!" or "Been there and done that," give this move a chance. This is not the same ol' sex-in-the-car bit. Think outside the four doors and do sex differently. Buckle up, road warriors. This will be one road trip he'll never forget.

The Move: Slinging Dixie (Sex in a Seat-Belt Sling)

You've probably seen sex slings online or in sex toy stores. This move plays on the idea, with the added thrill of doing it in a car. Having one or both legs lifted gives you incredible G-spot stimulation and offers him a fantastic view of your pussy.

THE PREPARATIONS
★ Dress for the part: no panties; no bra; a little sundress with a full skirt, a short flippy skirt with a tank top, or one of his button-down shirts and nothing else. Ask him to strip down to baggy shorts or swim trunks—or wrap a towel around his waist as he gets out of the shower. Clothing needs to be nonrestrictive and provide easy genital access.
★ Park the car in the garage—so the neighbors won't call the cops.

THE LEAD-IN

Tell him you're taking him on a virtual road trip. Blindfold him and slowly walk him to his car. Ask questions, like "What are you thinking about?" "Are you excited [as you touch his package]?" "Do you know where you are?"

Gently seat him in the backseat of the car. Turn on your favorite radio station. Reach over to put his seat belt on. On the return put your head in his lap.

THE FOREPLAY

① Put your mouth around his clothed penis and make a humming sound that comes from deep in your throat. This will send vibrations up and down his spine and give him something too yummy to think about for the next few minutes.

② Straddle him. Kiss his neck and ears. Bury his face in your breasts. With his blindfold still on, allow him to suckle and lick your nipples. Press your vulva against his cock.

③ When you get to a song that inspires you and makes you feel like the sensual woman you are, touch your pussy, stroke your clitoris, and feel your own excitement grow. Put your juicy fingers to his lips and share the love.

④ Remove his blindfold. Ask him if he's having flashbacks of getting off to hot rod magazine fantasies—beautiful babes on glossy pages in one hand, his cock in the other.

⑤ Unbuckle his seat belt and whisper, "I'm going to make those dreams come true for you."

SEX FACT

According to an MSNBC/*Elle* survey, couples who have good sexual communication and are open to trying new things in the bedroom also tend to be more satisfied with each other over the years.

THE SEXPERT SAYS

You have probably heard the saying "Couples who play together stay together." Sex is a symbolic act, which means that we can choose what it means to us and how we feel about it. The options and combinations are literally unlimited and go beyond the bed (or car).

★ The Main Act

1 Pull on your seat belt, the one closest to the passenger door, so you have plenty of slack. Weave the seat belt through that hook for your dry cleaning that you never use and have him lace up your ankles so your feet are bound but your legs are wide open in the shape of an O. The effect is similar to that created by a costly sex sling designed to lift your rear, giving your partner access to your genital hot spots.

2 He slides between your legs, with your feet and the seat belt resting across his upper back. Keep the door open so he has room to move and thrust deeply.

3 Grab his butt and pull his pelvis in to you.

♀ WHY IT WORKS FOR HER

★ The sling is amazing, mostly because you don't have to hold your legs up and can leverage your body in new and different ways. And this position allows you to relax, which means deeper, more comfortable penetration.

★ This angle affords excellent G-spot stimulation.

♂ WHY IT WORKS FOR HIM

★ Men love deep thrusting! And this position is visually stimulating and psychologically thrilling: you are surrendering to him with your legs wide open, waiting for his penetration. Offering him control of the sling is like handing over the remote.

★ Men crave variety in their sexual experiences—and this one gives him something he's never had before.

RELATED MOVES

★ Have him put a hand under your butt and lift you closer to him.

★ Put your hands over your head and grasp the top of the other passenger door so you can push your body toward him as he thrusts.

★ Sit in the middle of the seat, loop the seat-belt harness closest to each of the doors through the dry-cleaning handles, and put one leg in each of the loops. He positions in front of you for vaginal penetration and a great view of you spread-eagle. With this position, you can close the doors.

★ From the position above, you can switch so he can be the one in the sling and get a blow job and, if he's game, a P-spot massage. Nice!

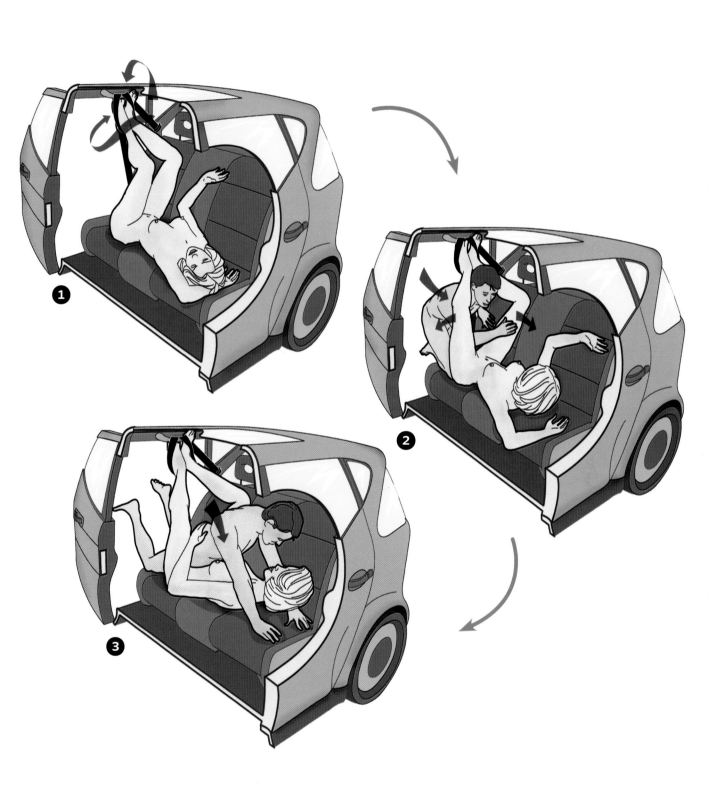

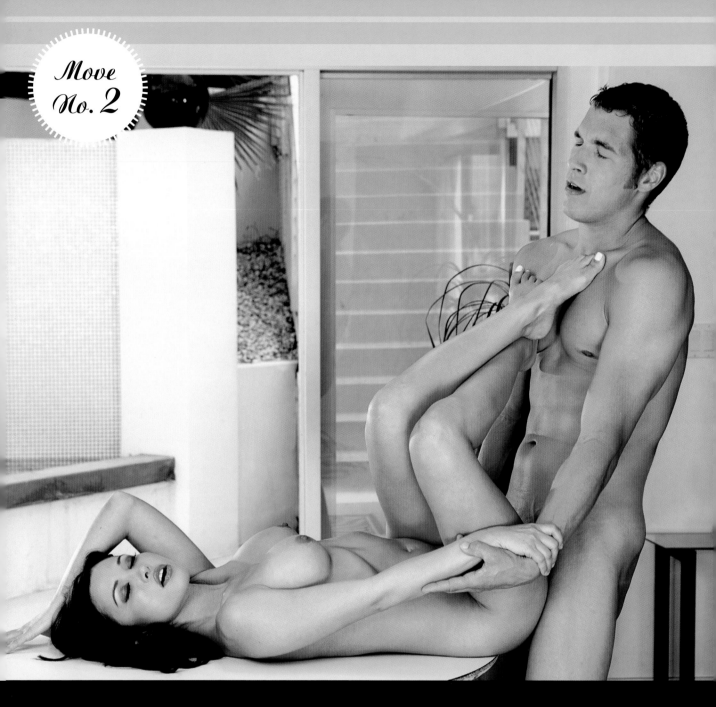

DINNER FOR TWO

With one swift swoop of the hand and without a second thought, push all those dishes off the table, letting them land where they may. Replace the old whispers of "Oh no, my floor!" with

The Move: Dinner for Two

THE PREPARATIONS

★ Pull out those cute, summery plastic dishes, even if it's winter, and set your table.

★ You don't have to actually put food on the plates, but if you must, think "easy to vacuum or sweep" types of foods like raw veggies (no dressing) or pretzels.

★ If you are like most women, you are going to need to practice this one. Throwing things on the floor is totally counterintuitive. We have been trained to pick things up, not consciously throw them on the floor.

★ You will probably hear that little voice in your head saying, "Don't do that." Put on your finest underwear and tell that otherwise helpful little voice, "It's plastic and I can clean it up in the morning." (Maybe he will even be cleaning it up after this move.)

THE LEAD-IN

The next time you dine together, take a bite of your food or sip of your wine and let the appreciation show without ever saying a word. Use what you've got to say, "This is delicious."

Get up and walk around the table to him. Facing him, put your hands on his shoulders, look him in the eye, and order him: "Fuck me now, on the table."

Disclaimer: Not recommended for glass, wicker, or other unstable tables.

THE FOREPLAY

① Keep up a hot-and-heavy pace with heavy breathing and panting. Quickly remove your panties. Kiss him, but if you have to break mouth contact once in a while, hold the eye gaze.

THE SEXPERT SAYS

Most of us want to share intimate or sexy thoughts and feelings with our lover, but how do we do it without feeling silly? You will probably feel really silly at first. As always, you need to practice.

To make it easy, describe what you Feel, Imagine, or Think. The acronym is FIT. I Feel my heart beat quickly whenever you touch me. When we were in the parking lot yesterday, I Imagined what it would be like for you to put me on the hood of your truck, lift up my dress, and have your way with me. I am on my lunch hour right now and I can't stop Thinking about your perfect cock and the way you feel inside me.

Use FIT with other positions (such as Mutual Masturbation Play-by-Play) that give you a lot of practice saying what you are experiencing.

★ The Main Act

1 Lie on your back and spread your legs open, keeping them flat on the table to start.

2 Ask him to get on top of you on the table in man-on-top (missionary) position.

3 Because you are both so turned on, you will be able to sustain this position on the table for a little longer than usual.

4 When it's time to switch, scoot down toward the end of the table so that your butt is at the edge and he is standing. Guide him into helping by putting his hands on your legs, indicating he should grab hold and pull you into him.

5 Make him swoon while he is thrusting by lifting your lusty legs to the left, right, crossing them, putting them over his shoulder—whatever feels good. Explore the feelings.

6 At some point, bend your legs at the knees and pull them against your chest. He grasps your buttocks as he thrusts from the standing position.

7 Push and pull your way to orgasm with this edgy move.

♀ WHY IT WORKS FOR HER

★ This is a hot and empowering move and, in the end, a great exercise in turning off that little voice that gets in the way of sex. How many times have you ruined an otherwise perfectly sexy moment by straightening the pillows or closing drawers and doors?

♂ WHY IT WORKS FOR HIM

★ Your razor-sharp focus to fuck him and reckless abandonment of the plasticware is hot! Girl, you have just earned the "Best He's Ever Had" award. Heck, you're probably the best lover you ever had.

RELATED MOVES

★ Lie on your stomach and hang your ass over the edge of the table. In this position he has full access to your G-spot.

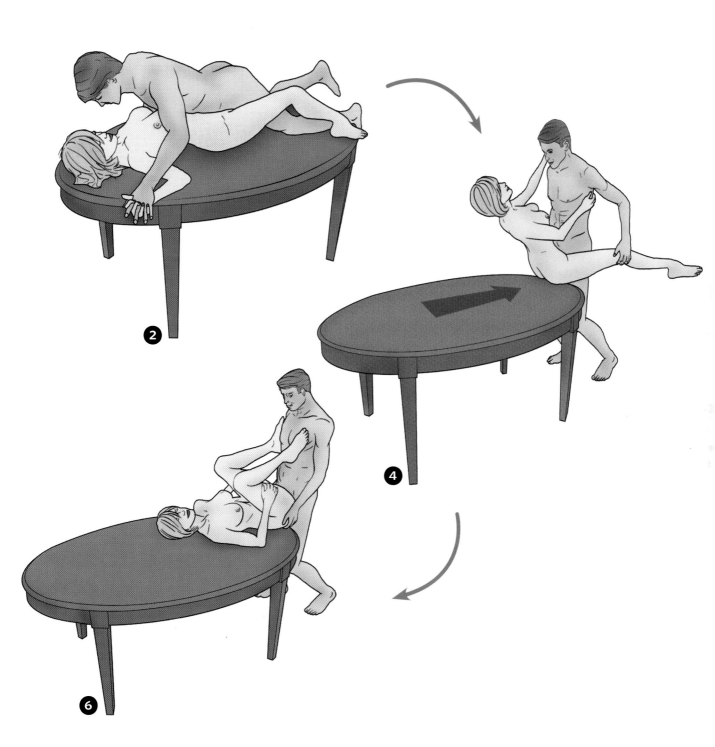

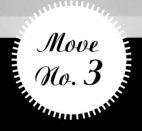

Move No. 3

SPRING FEVER

Has the playfulness gone out of your relationship and been replaced with predictability? Is fun zapped by worries of how to pay the bills? Everyone needs to bust loose and have a break from responsibilities, even if just for a moment. Help him to take a mental vacation and get back in touch with his playful little boy.

The Move: Spring Fever

Picture this: On the slide in your own backyard, lay on your back with legs spread open. He straddles your body on the slide. As he thrusts, you will slide down, allowing for deeper penetration. He can control depth by holding your position with his hands on your hips.

THE PREPARATIONS

★ **Finally:** a good use for a piece of neglected outdoor play equipment! Clean off the slide in your backyard. Wear a skirt and tank top and no underwear.

★ **Do this at night**—with the outdoor lights off.

THE LEAD-IN

Put on your girlish charm and ask him if he can come out and play with you. If he seems hesitant or insists that he has to work or wants to watch TV, lift up your top and flash your chest. When you get his yes, guide him to the slide.

Disclaimer: Make sure you use the slide in your own backyard.

THE FOREPLAY

① Get into the spirit of the play by going down the slide a few times. Feel the long-lost freedom of playfulness.

② Lead him to your backyard side and go up the ladder. If he hasn't noticed you aren't wearing panties, turn around, give him your girlish smile, cover your ass, and say, "No peeking." Of course he will look.

③ When you are behind him on the way up the ladder, rub your breasts into his back. Reach in front and rub his cock through his clothing.

SEX FACTS

• A 2008 *Cosmopolitan*/Durex survey reports that 32.7 percent of the respondents say that exhaustion or stress keeps them from having sex more often.

• Psychologists estimate that 15 to 20 percent of couples have sex no more than ten times a year.

THE SEXPERT SAYS

Many male clients who come in to see me are talking about the good ol' days and questioning their desire for their partner, when the real issue is usually stress and overworking, leaving no time for fun, play, or pleasure. Sex is all of these things. So, when sex is no longer a part of the picture or holds little or no importance between people, many are left wondering what happened. Doing Spring Fever will help bring you back to the good ol' days and put the fun back into sex.

⭐ *The Main Act*

1 Start by sitting upright on the slide, face forward toward your man. He is waiting at the end of the slide. Lie on your back with your legs spread open and arms extended. Hold onto the bars at the top of the slide as you wait to slip down.

2 Standing mid-slide, he spreads his legs so one leg is on each side of the slide and the chute runs between.

3 Push your feet against the inside of the slide and use them as your brakes on the way down so you have control and can stop. Let your arms go and inch your way down to his penis for a nice sliding penetration. He will likely have to put his hands to the side of the slide and lean his upper body into you.

4 As he thrusts, begin to "release the brakes"—in other words, stop pushing your feet against the insides of the slide. He can now control the depth of penetration by holding your position with his hands on your hips and lifting you up and down. Tilt your pelvis upward to hit your clitoris and G-spot.

5 If you have to hold your position in the inside of the slide, it will require you to tighten muscles in your lower body, which helps make for a more sensational orgasm.

♀ WHY IT WORKS FOR HER

★ You are in control of the depth and degree of penetration, so this position frees him of the burden to perform and allows him to enjoy you enjoying him.

♂ WHY IT WORKS FOR HIM

★ Not only are you giving him a momentary mental vacation, but you are also relieving him of the burden of performing sexually by initiating and guiding this position.

RELATED MOVES

★ For a new sensation, lift a leg and put your foot to his chest. Tilt your pelvis for positioning.

★ Push your legs together and close them tightly for a snug fit around his penis.

★ When he is in increased arousal mode, turn over on your knees so your ass is facing him and your hands holding on to the sides of the slides. Release your weight as he pulls you onto his cock and thrusts into a spring-feverish orgasm.

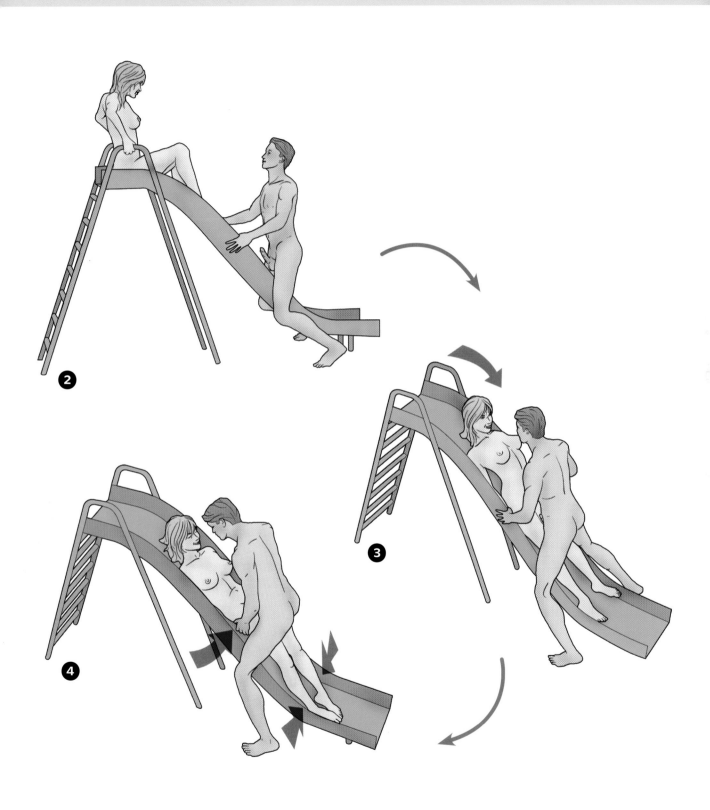

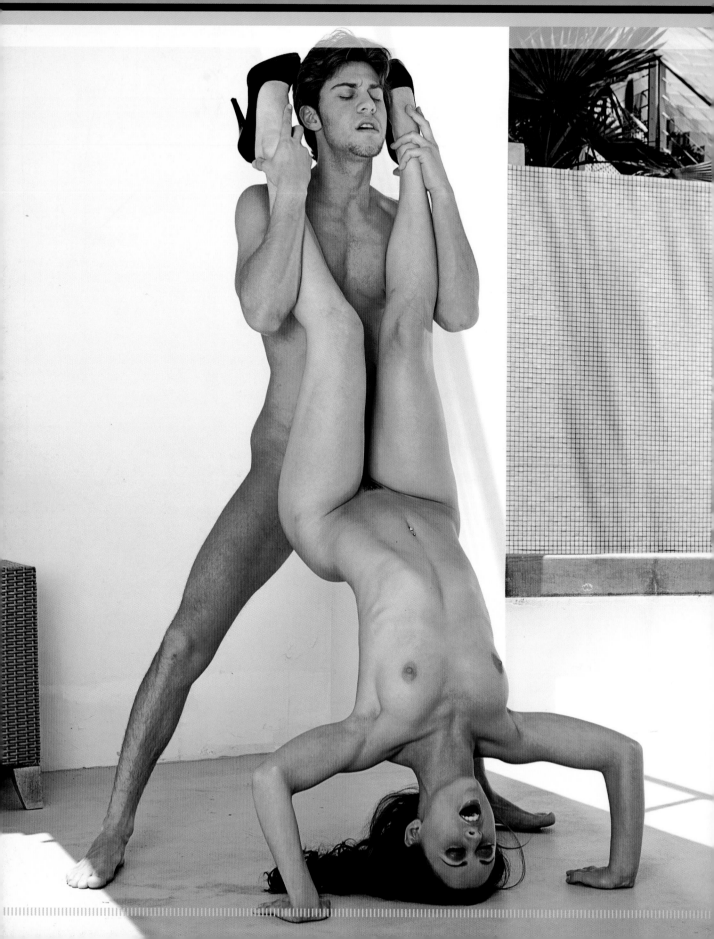

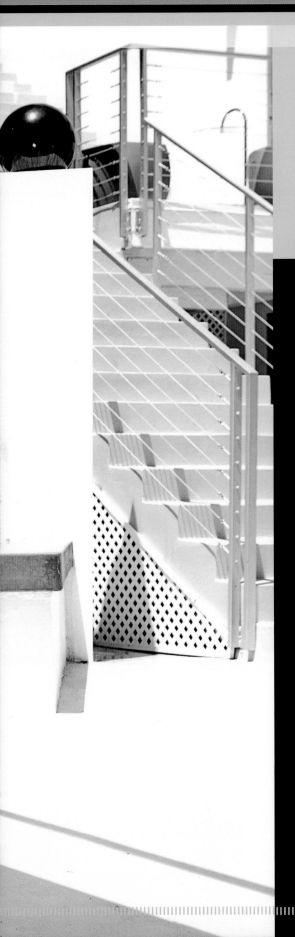

Rear Entry

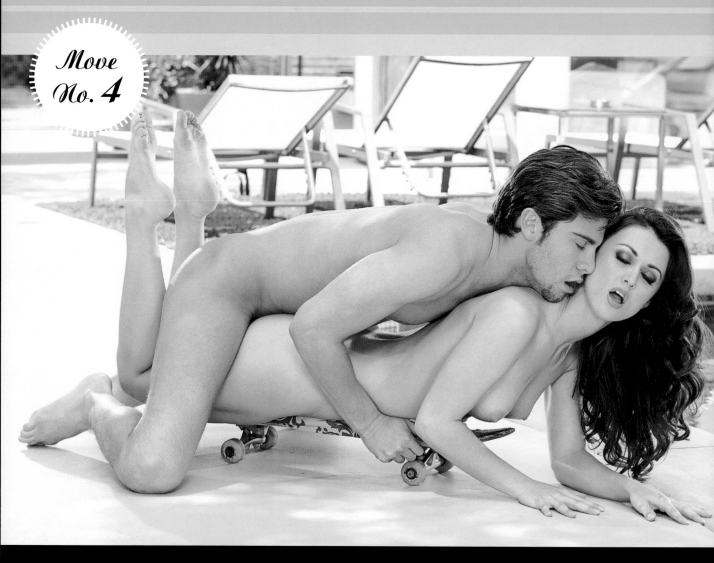

Move No. 4

★ HEAD OVER WHEELS

If sex is lying on your belly and moving your butt forward and backward, it still gets boring for you and tiring for him.

The perfect solution is to add wheels. You lie on your stomach on a skateboard. After inserting his penis, he pulls you in from behind. Gliding intercourse—with no rug burn. Brilliant.

The Move: Head Over Wheels

THE PREPARATIONS

★ Locate a skateboard. It doesn't have to be high quality unless, of course, you have a sponsor or are doing sexy tricks.

★ Find a smooth, flat, and hard surface that the skateboard can roll on. This move will not work on thick carpet, but it will work on wood, tile, or thinly carpeted floors. You don't need a lot of room because you are not actually going to ride it, but you will need to have room to lie down on the board.

★ Put your hair up—you don't want it to get run over. Ouch!

★ Lie naked on the skateboard on your belly and take it for a trial spin. Need pillows? If yes, lay down a thin pillow that is comfy and fits the size of the board. Grab one for his knees, too—or pull out the kneepads from your sports days.

THE LEAD-IN

Find your man and roll out naked on the skateboard. Sit on the skateboard, knees bent, and roll it toward and away from him. When you roll it toward him, open your legs for a nice bird's-eye view. When you pull away close your legs a little, adding anticipation to the fun.

Ask him if he can come out to play. Skateboarding has been around since the 1950s, however, I can almost guarantee you that will be his first Head Over Wheels vixen.

THE FOREPLAY

① Tell him that if he wants to skate with you, he must be naked; It's a trendy California thing.

② First the warm-up: ask him to lie down with his back on the board, facing the ceiling.

③ You are sitting on your knees, looking at his body in the horizontal position, with your head directly above his penis, one hand under his body at the front of the board, and the other hand on the back of the board.

④ Stick out your tongue, bend over to his penis, and move the board back and forth, to and fro.

⑤ Turn your head to the left or right so that when you move the board back and forth, his penis goes in and out, your mouth acting like a tunnel.

⑥ Now hover over him with your butt over his face and look down on his penis. If you were to lie down on him, you would be in the 69 position with you on top.

⑦ Lean down, open your mouth, and begin moving the board again. Go slowly for precision. If you miss your mouth while going slowly, it won't hurt him.

⑧ Now add a little suction so he can really feel it.

⑨ When you glide the penis out of your mouth, purse your lips closed, so he can feel your lips on the head of his penis, the most sensitive spot.

⭐ The Main Act

1 Help him off the board and then lie down with your belly to the board, using pillows as needed. Your butt should just be hanging over the back end of the board, so scoot down or forward for optimal positioning.

2 Place a pillow on the floor for his knees.

3 Spread your legs and ask him to enter you. Direct him to lean over you on all fours and insert his cock into your pussy (or penis into vagina, whatever terms you prefer).

4 Put your hands on the ground and glide your body back and forth, and thus his penis in and out. Start slowly and increase the speed as you both get into the body-boarding rhythm.

♀ WHY IT WORKS FOR HER

★ You're just rolling, baby. This is a no-effort position. Perfect for those days you want to be fun and playful but are just too tired to think up something.

♂ WHY IT WORKS FOR HIM

★ This position is sexy because it suggests that you see a world of erotic opportunities all around you and in everyday items. Voilà—something in common. You are teasing him by putting your butt in the air, moving it toward and away from him, luring him in. Anytime wheels and a naked woman's body are involved, it's a hot ride. He will love the ease with which he can roll you and control the penetration and move you in and out for deeper thrusts.

RELATED MOVES

★ Lie on your back on the board with your feet to your shoulders. He moves you by the thighs. He needs to be skillful for this move. You'll want to use a pillow.

★ You lie on your belly on the board with your butt raised while he squats. This is particularly useful if you don't have a pillow handy for his knees. Again, make sure you push back.

★ While you lie on your belly, open your legs a bit so he can put his knees between yours, on the inside. Again, raise your butt and push backward and forward.

★ Do the same as in the position above, but in this variation, he puts his knees on the outside.

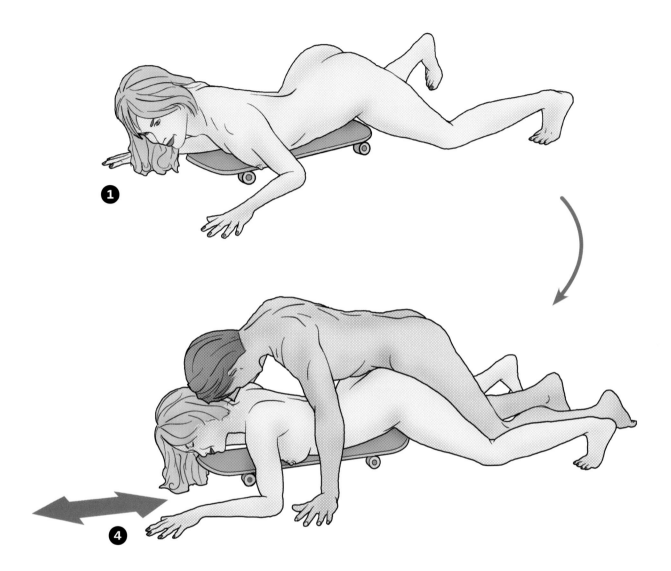

||||||||||||||||||||||||||||||||||||||||||||||||||||||||||||||||||||||||||||||||||||||||||||||||||||||||||||||||||||||||||||||||||||||||||||||||||||||

SEX FACT

Fifty- three percent of men who responded to an MSNBC/*Elle* survey said they felt more desired by their partners in the early days of the relationship.

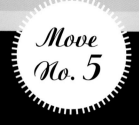

MIRROR IMAGES

Up the sexual ante with this move. Do it standing in front of a dresser mirror. Lean forward, putting your weight on your hands, as he enters from behind.

The Move: Mirror Images

THE PREPARATIONS

★ Accessorize! Go shopping for fun little things that you can wear under your clothes to feel sexy and that will also make a generous gift to your lover that evening. For example, beads or pearls are beautiful and they can be wrapped around his cock for an exceptional blow job. (For more details on mind-blowing BJs, read my book *Oral Sex He'll Never Forget*.) Other ideas include sparkly lotions, garter belts, remote-control panties, clip-on navel jewelry, press-on tattoos, or anything that he can touch, taste, or smell and that will send him straight to Orgasmville.

THE LEAD-IN

You and your reflection are sexual dynamos. Let him see you slowly undressing in the mirror, feeling sexual and sensual.

Start the sensual moves from the head and work your way down to your toes. Run your fingers through your hair, lifting it off your shoulders. Glide your fingers from your ear down to the perky nipples of your breasts and let out a moan of pleasure.

Slowly remove your shirt and your bra, loving what you see in the mirror. Sexy thoughts fill your mind as you remove your panties.

If he did not look up when you moaned, try moaning louder. If he still doesn't notice, involve him in the mirror play by asking him to put lotion on you.

When you are fully naked or wearing only your thigh-high stockings and high heels, bend down at the waist, as if looking for something.

Once he is in mirror view, tell him how you like to see him touching you. Be authentic and true when you tell him what you like.

THE FOREPLAY

① Look in the mirror and watch how you inspire feelings of desire, attraction, significance, and safety.

② Using the lotion or oil, touch your vulva, nipples, ass, or anyplace that gives you pleasure. Make sure whatever lotion or oil you use is sex-friendly so there are no limits to where the play can go.

③ Stick out your butt, reach through your legs, separate your labia, and invite him in.

THE SEXPERT SAYS

Lingerie is a flag that you wave to send signals to his brain that you got dressed up and beautiful because you want sex with him. But lingerie in itself is not sexiness. In fact, the actual definition is "women's underwear"; basically, it is just material. But how you *feel* and what you bring to the material with your sensuality and confidence is what turns ordinary underwear into something hot.

★ The Main Act

1 Ask him to be inside of you, to fuck or penetrate you, or however you prefer to phrase your request. Notice that first moment of insertion when he enters you.

2 Tilt your pelvis up and down to find what feels good.

3 Put your legs together for a more snug fit. If he pulls his penis all the way out, he will get the sensation on the head of his cock all the way down his shaft when he reenters.

4 Widen your stance and spread your legs open for a looser fit. He will feel the sensation more on the underside of his penis.

5 Power your booty by moving it forward and backward, receiving and resisting him. Extend your arms to offer more resistance, and move in the direction of his thrusts to receive him.

6 Contract your PC muscles to grip the shaft of his penis. Bear down a bit to give a looser feeling. Bearing down usually adds sensation to the head and makes him thrust faster and harder in fear of being ejected from the vagina.

7 Find a rhythm, contracting, tilting, and thrusting your way to orgasm.

♀ WHY IT WORKS FOR HER

★ Unobstructed access to your G-spot and your hands free to rub your clit earns this position the first choice award.

♂ WHY IT WORKS FOR HIM

★ He can see your bodacious rear, your bouncing breasts, and your gorgeous face all in the same glance as he goes deliciously deep inside of you.

RELATED MOVES

★ Take a few steps back from the mirror and turn to face him sitting on the bed. With no panties, in high heels, keep your legs straight as you bend at the waist to put his cock in your mouth. To give him a sensational mirror show, wear a really short skirt that draws his eyes further and further up your skirt with each dip down deep to the back of your throat. This variation will give him a look at himself being pleasured and a good view of your high-heeled, lengthened legs.

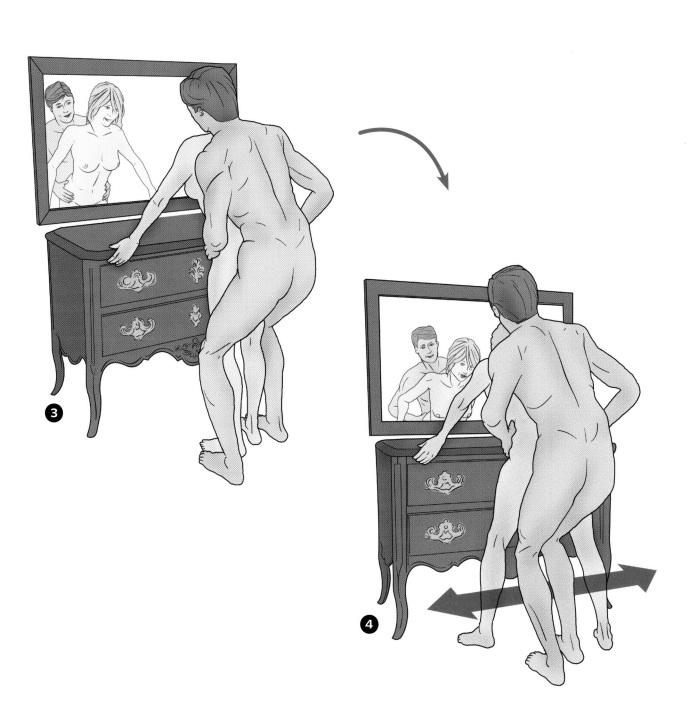

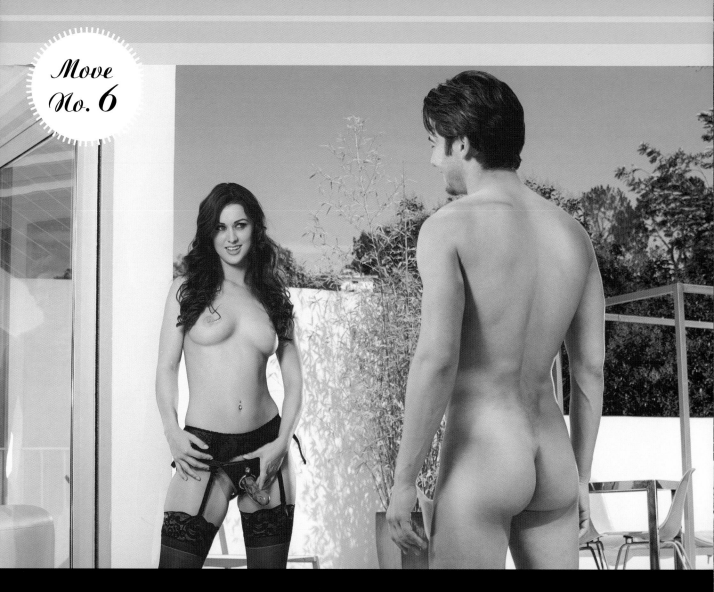

FLOWER POWER

Give him the gift of being penetrated and let him experience the feeling of fullness.
Wielding a strap-on requires special considerations and skills that you may not have yet.
Now's the time to learn how.

 Using a dildo and a harness is a great way to stimulate his prostate, also fondly known
as the P-spot. Penetration and being penetrated is about more than just hitting the right spots;
it is emotionally erotic and may lead to orgasm all on its own.

The Move: Flower Power

THE PREPARATIONS

If you don't already have a strap-on and dildo, visit a sex toy store (or a good website like Babeland.com) to get information about how to choose the right products for you and your partner.

★ Make sure you use plenty of lube for both comfort and safety. The anus does not lubricate naturally, at least not enough for penetration. It can tear easily, which is not only painful, but could also be a gateway for infection. A water-based lube works best with a condom. Condoms are ideal for easy cleanup. Do not share your dildo or go from vagina to anus.

★ For additional information and inspiration, watch the video *Bend Over Boyfriend*.

THE LEAD-IN

You can initiate the Flower Power position in different ways. Try pointing out a strap-on at a sex toy store, or watch a video together and ask, "Hey, would you like to try that with me?" Or you could just flat-out tell him what you would like to do with him.

THE FOREPLAY

① Take a warm bath together. This will relax him, and the conversation you have can give him added confidence before anal play.

② Create safety in the bathtub and build anticipation for the act by talking about penetrating him. Discuss what's exciting about it for you.

③ Position yourselves so he is lying in the tub with his legs open and you are sitting between his legs and facing him. Rest a soapy finger at the base of his anus and gently press down so your finger slides in easily (never force your finger or any object into the anus).

④ Bend your finger at the knuckle and make the "come hither" motion toward you. You should feel a firm, bulbous tissue that might feel a lot like the tip of your nose. This is the prostate. Rub that in different ways to see what feels good to your partner.

⑤ Then get out of the bath, towel him dry, and take him to the bed.

⑥ Strap on your dildo. Touch and feel it. Let him play with it and suck it if he wants to.

⑦ Position him on all fours, while you get on your knees directly behind him. Another similar position is to have him bend over, holding on to a chair or table, while you stand. Without insertion, gently lay your body weight over him and lead him into some deep breaths.

★ The Main Act

1 Put some lube on your hand, reach over, and manually stimulate his cock. This will feel good and help relax him.

2 You can kiss his back and butt cheeks, or if you enjoy rimming, place a piece of plastic wrap over his butthole and go to town.

3 When you notice him becoming aroused and relaxed, remove any plastic wrap and apply plenty of lube to the tip of the dildo and to his anus. Gently press down at the base of his anus so the dildo slides in easily just as you did with your finger in the bathtub. If you find him still difficult to penetrate, do more oral sex, have vaginal sex, or begin penetrating him with something smaller, like a plug or your finger.

4 Go slowly and have a gradual build. Never force anything in. Ask him if it's okay before going faster or deeper. Stay in communication with him so you can take him to soaring heights. Remember, your responsibility as the penetrator is to develop trust.

5 When the time is right to switch, pull out just as slowly and try another position:

★ **The Bucking Bronco:** You lie down on your back, while he sits on top and rides you like a bull.

★ **The Capricorn:** You sit on your feet with your knees bent. Hold him while he sits on top of the dildo.

★ **Spooning:** He lies in front of you while you hold him from behind. Tilt your pelvis up and let him wiggle and shake onto the dildo.

★ **Froggy:** He squats onto your dildo while you sit on a chair or couch. Make sure he has the chairback or something to hold on to as he lowers and raises onto you.

6 Make up your own positions, have fun, and be creative with the Flower Power move as you take him where no ordinary orgasm can.

♀ WHY IT WORKS FOR HER

★ Many women feel empowered by penetrating a man. It also helps to develop an understanding of the level of trust that is required to penetrate a loved one. You might also see a softness emerge in him that you haven't noticed in the other positions you have tried.

♂ WHY IT WORKS FOR HIM

★ He will discover what is emotionally required to be penetrated.

RELATED MOVES

★ Choose a dildo that adds vibration to your clitoris.

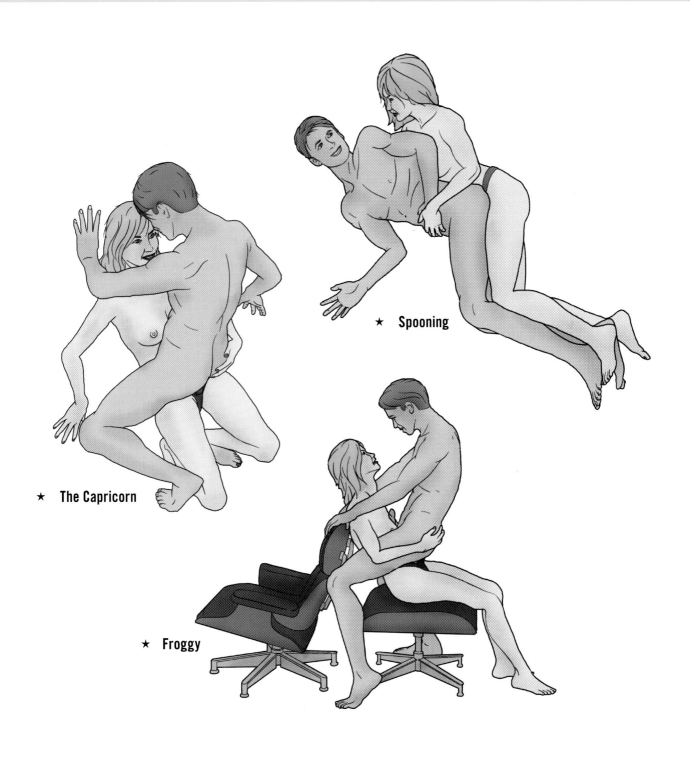

★ Spooning

★ The Capricorn

★ Froggy

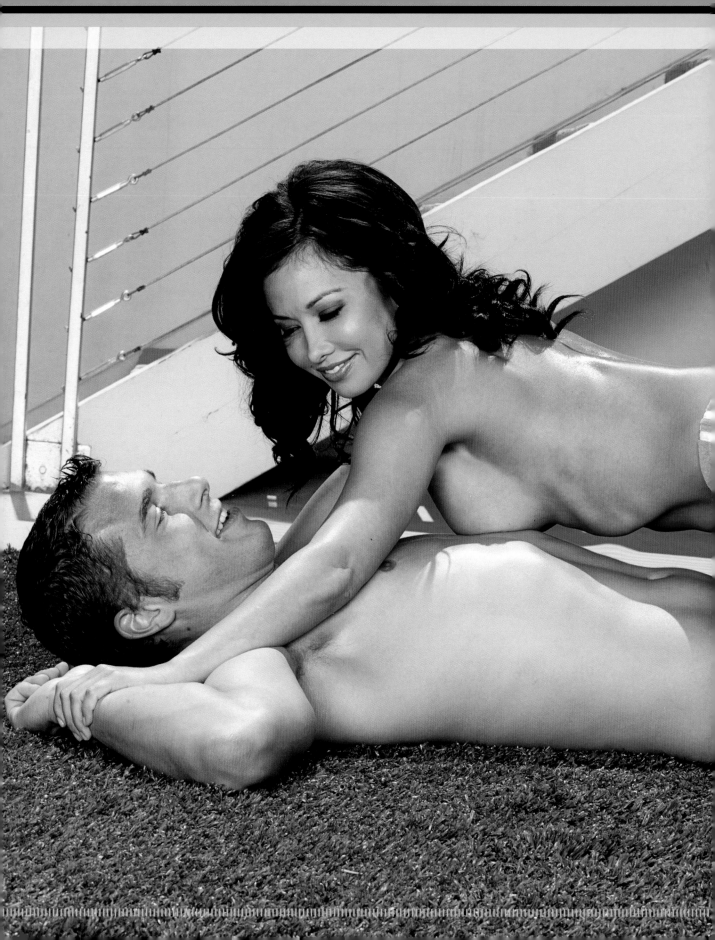

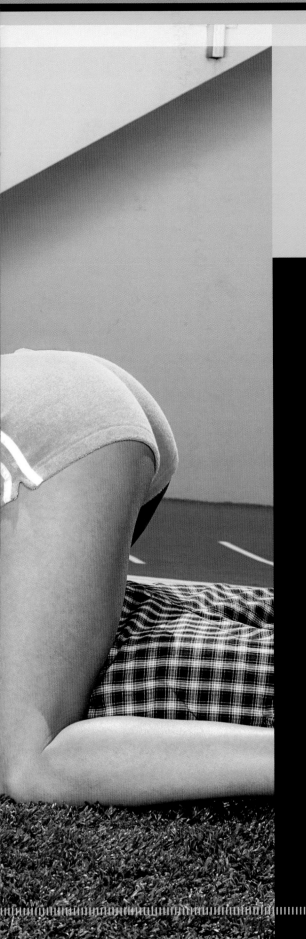

She's on Top

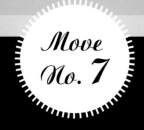

THE STIMULUS PLAN

Sometimes there is conflict, and sometimes the best path to conflict resolution is to wrestle it out under the sheets. Grease up and wrestle out your negative energies naked. Have him lie flat on his back and pin him down so he can't get up as you grind your clitoris against his pelvic bone before you ride him.

The Move: The Stimulus Plan

THE PREPARATIONS

★ Put a sheet that you don't care about getting dirty on the carpet. Set out two bottles of massage oil (jojoba is amazing for the skin), one in his corner and one in yours, and then turn on the heater.

★ For added fun, play the "Eye of the Tiger" song—clearly another boxing reference, but who cares! It's worth a laugh and you need a little lightness right now.

★ Agree on a "tap out" term and gesture. When one of you hits the floor with your hand or yells out a random, agreed-upon word like "Cheerios," you need to put all contact to a halt because someone got hurt.

★ Listen up: this is your coach talking here. You likely won't win this match with your brawn, so you will need a strategy. You are going to rely on your feminine graces. Your feminine graces have an incredible power—power that all of the great goddesses used to launch ships and cause men to forget their own names. You have that power, and today you will use it.

★ Don't worry. I'll also give you technique.

THE LEAD-IN

Walk up to him naked, hand him a bottle of massage oil, and tell him that you want to resolve this with a wrestling match.

THE FOREPLAY

① Stand across from him as if you were opponents on opposite sides of the ring, lathering up for your match and talking dirtier than you ever have before. Remember that your bark is bigger than your bite, and that's okay here.

② Lather your arms, legs, and oh-so-beautiful breasts with the oil. While you're oiling up your breasts, you may as well enjoy it and let him see you enjoying yourself: twist those nipples.

③ Your silly wrestling boy may try to intimidate with his scary faces, but you are making him weak with your beauty before you even make contact. This is important, so don't hold back here: moan, squeal, squirm, shake with pleasure. If you do, he has no chance.

||||||||||||||||||||||||||||||||||||||||||||||||||||||||||||||||||||||||||||||||||||||||||||||||||||||||||||||||||

SEX FACT

According to the *Cosmopolitan*/Durex survey, 30 percent of respondents said that an argument with their partners ruined their libido.

||||||||||||||||||||||||||||||||||||||||||||||||||||||||||||||||||||||||||||||||||||||||||||||||||||||||||||||||||

THE SEXPERT SAYS

It is normal to have conflict with someone. This is particularly true in matters of sex and intimacy, where we are our most vulnerable. Issues come up, but neither the nature of the conflict nor the end result is as important as the process. There are many different ways to handle any one situation—millions, I'd imagine. But most often, time and time again, we will do what we have always done. Not because what we've always done has worked or because it is the best solution, but simply because it's what we are comfortable with. Try something new, something playful.

★ The Main Act

1 Reach your arm out to shake hands, and when you make contact, gently pull him close to you and reach your other hand out to quickly stroke his cock.

2 Oil him up, killing him with kindness.

3 Take him to the bed and have him lie on his stomach. Give him a relaxing massage, soothing all of that tightness built up from the argument. Tell him to take deep breaths and release all the tension. Muscle memory is the strongest form of memory, so really get that stuff out.

4 Turn him over onto his back. Liberally add oil to the front of his body, using much more than what you would use for a normal massage. Give him a few long strokes and then proceed to lather yourself with the oil. Again, use much more than you would normally. Add plenty of lube to his cock. Rub it with long strokes to achieve the desired firmness.

5 Before insertion, you are going to get him into a sexy pin-down. Lie on top of him and weave your arms under his forearms and then over his palms. Starting on the outside, weave your legs under his knees and bring your feet over the calves. SLOWLY extend your arms and legs. Congratulations! You pinned him! He didn't see that one coming.

6 After celebrating, lie on top of him with your legs slightly open and slip slide away. For a more snug fit, close your legs.

7 Bring him in on the action by asking him to grip your ass and glide it up and down his cock to orgasm.

♀ WHY IT WORKS FOR HER

★ Stop doing what doesn't work, change the climate, and have great sex.

♂ WHY IT WORKS FOR HIM

★ This move gives him a new perspective on you, and on "fighting" in general.

RELATED MOVES

★ Switch so he is on top of you as you lie on your back doing nothing. And I mean nothing, except receiving him. Watch him take over and maneuver you into creative positions.

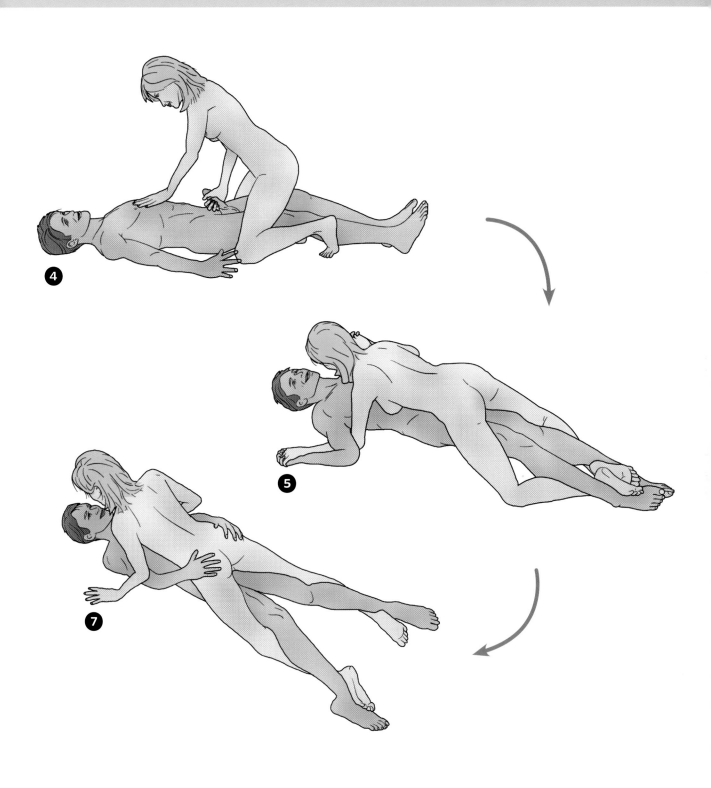

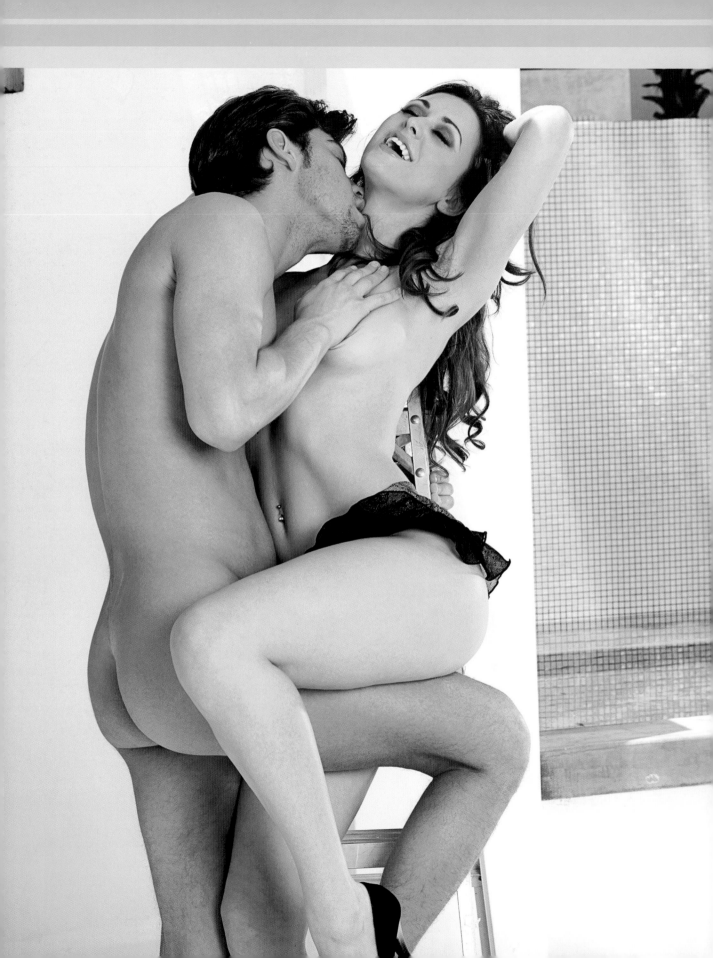

SHOOTS <u>AND</u> LADDERS

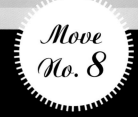

When did you last use that fire escape ladder? Or the ladder that leads up to the backyard playground slide? The gift of a great sex life is seeing and acting in the moment.

The Move: Shoots and Ladders

THE PREPARATIONS

★ You must wear a skirt, without panties—unless, of course, you are in a secluded place or don't care about prancing around without any bottoms.

★ And choose your ladder wisely. Public play can be exciting and highly erotic, but there can be legal ramifications, so be discreet.

★ *Note:* Only use attached, stable ladders that are safe and secure.

THE LEAD-IN

Guide him to the ladder. Lean onto it, raise your hands above your head, look him in the eye, and tell him you would like to feel him penetrating you. Whisper in his ear that you could get a lot of depth, a good fuck, using the ladder.

THE FOREPLAY

① While still holding the ladder, bend your knees and rub your body against his.

② Tell him how aroused you are—for example, that you are slippery wet, and put his finger inside you. Wrap your legs around him and move your hips in a little bump and grind or "outercourse."

⭐ *The Main Act*

1 Climb up a few steps on the ladder. How many depends on how much taller he is. Slowly ease down onto his cock (while simultaneously working your quads!).

2 When you get to the base of his cock, move your pelvis back and forth and side to side.

3 Allow him to hear your sounds. When he hits a place that feels good, let it be known. Moan and sigh as you need to.

4 Contract your PC muscles on the upstrokes, gripping his penis much like he does with his hand on the upstroke when he masturbates. When you are up and out of him, rub your wet pussy over the head of his cock. The head is very sensitive, and men will often rub their hand over it on the upstroke when masturbating.

5 Maintain slow thrusting for as long as you can. You can always speed up, but like the clit, the cock can become desensitized quickly and it doesn't feel as good to slow down again. If he starts taking control and lifting and lowering your ass in an effort to go faster, tell him to take it slow or place his hands where you want them. For example, whisper in his ear, telling him to stimulate your nipples, his nipples, his own ass, or his balls. Your directing makes this move feel so fresh and erotic.

6 Straddle him so he is holding your ass and raising and lowering you onto his cock. Raise your arms above you in surrender, clasping the ladder rungs for support and helping adjust the depth of penetration.

♀ WHY IT WORKS FOR HER

★ You control the depth of penetration by bending and extending your legs.

★ This position also gives him easier and more direct access to your cervix. Some women report that stimulation to the anterior (AFE zone) and posterior fornices surrounding the cervix creates an intense orgasm and an emotional release. Other women report that the fornices can't be stimulated without contact to the cervix, which might be painful at times and arousing at others. The fornices have been described as ringlike structures that encircle the cervix, with the texture similar to the back of a Frisbee.

★ Finally, there is less effort and fatigue because you are using the major muscles of your legs and arms.

♂ WHY IT WORKS FOR HIM

★ He loves see you taking your own pleasure.

RELATED MOVES

★ Turn around and hold onto the ladder so he enters from behind and you lower and raise yourself onto his cock at your own pace.

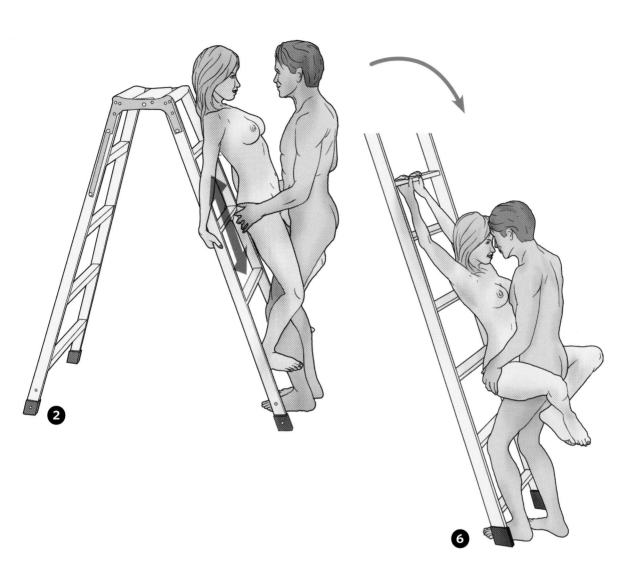

THE SEXPERT SAYS

A good way to talk dirty is to describe your own sexual arousal. Tell him how wet your pussy is, how erect your nipples are, or how engorged your clit is. Tell him what you think about when you see him eating your pussy or when you masturbated.

Only say this if it is true. If it is not true, ask yourself why you haven't allowed yourself to think sex-related thoughts.

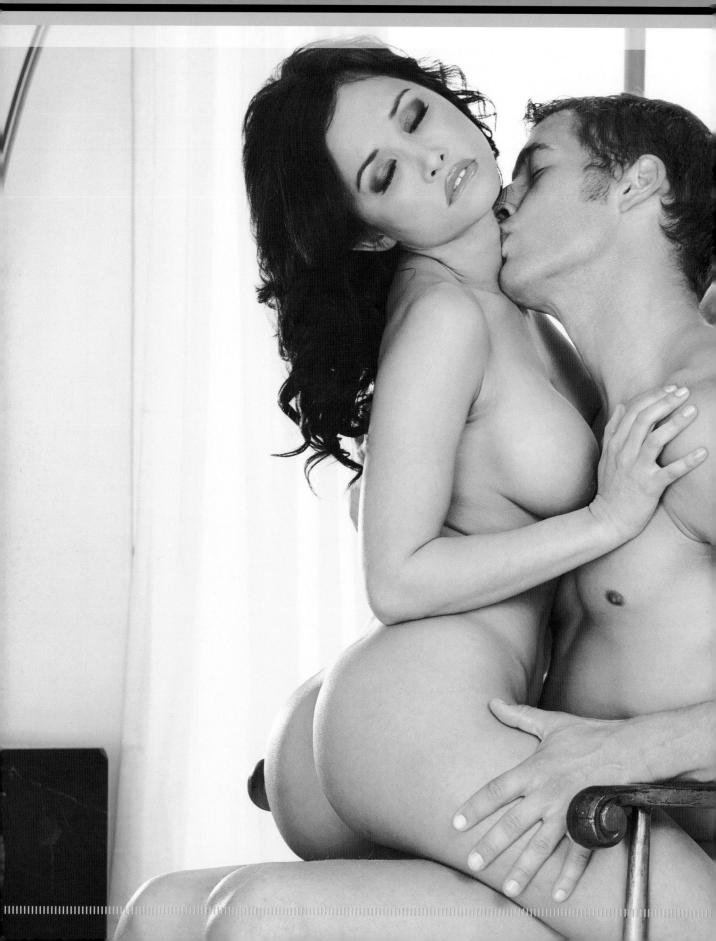

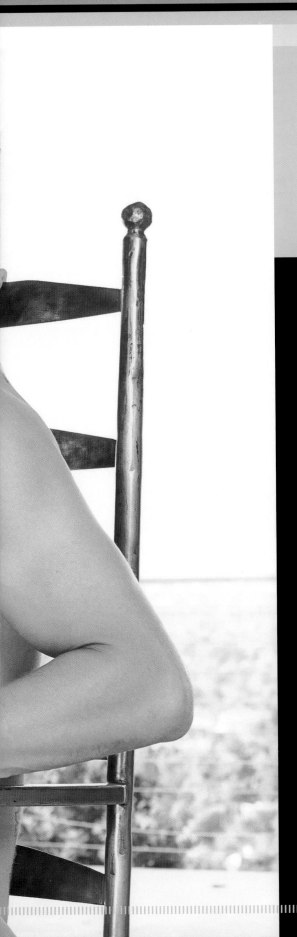

Sitting

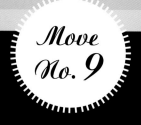

Move
No. 9

THE HARD ROCK

Rocking chairs are not just for grandmothers who knit. Sit on his lap and rock as he thrusts.

The Move: The Hard Rock

THE PREPARATIONS

★ Get a rocking chair. Set aside a few extra pillows to use as needed. (It's much easier to remove the pillows than it is to go searching for them when you are rocking and rolling.)

★ Put a coffee table or glider close by to rest your feet on. It will allow for leverage and some extra moves

★ For practice, push the rocker up to a table. You will need this for balance.

★ Imagine that he is in the chair and that you will straddle him with your legs spread, knees bent, and feet on the seat of the chair. So, your right foot is up against his left butt cheek and your left foot is up against his right butt cheek.

★ Practice tilting your pelvis back and forth, and moving it in circles. Have fun finding rhythms and patterns. There is no way to mess up.

THE LEAD-IN

Lead him to the ole rockin' chair and hold eye contact while you throw the knitting aside.

Remove his shoes and massage his shoulders. Just when he thinks he is getting a nice massage in grandma's chair, give him something naughty he didn't expect.

THE FOREPLAY

① Continue massaging him. Each time you massage an area, remove his clothing in that area. Turn it sexual by sucking, licking, and groaning. Think sexy thoughts and they will naturally be expressed in your touch.

② Massage his feet and take off his socks; massage his shoulders and remove his shirt; massage his legs and remove his pants; massage his cock and remove his underwear.

③ Now it is your turn to remove your clothing. Do it with a little flair: show him some shoulder and then cover it up. Remove your panties, bend over in just your skirt, and show him your ass. Lean in to kiss him, but don't and rub your chest up to his until your nipples reach his lips.

|||||||||||||||||||||||||||||||||||||||||||||||||||||||||||||||||||||||||||||||||||||||||||||||||||||||||||||||||||||||||||||||||

SEX FACT OR FICTION?

The Tang dynasty empress Wu-hou (who ruled from 683 to 705 AD) insisted that all visiting male dignitaries pay her homage by performing oral sex on her.

⭐ *The Main Act*

1 Straddle him with your legs spread, knees bent, and feet on the seat of the chair (your right foot against his left butt cheek and your left foot against his right butt cheek).

2 Place one hand behind the chair and one hand on the table for balance.

3 Start off simply sitting face to face. This is very sensual. To help get you started, connect with the eyes and match each other's breath.

4 Insert his penis into your vagina, flexing your PC muscle to hold it inside while you adjust with the pillows, etc. Just be together and rock and roll, finding your own rhythm.

5 When you want to switch positions, sit on his cock with your back to him. He pushes from the floor and back, you lean forward as though you're on a seesaw, a sexy seesaw.

6 In either position—facing him or with your back to him—he holds on to the arm of the chair and rocks it back and forth. He can control the angle and depth of penetration with the swing of the chair. This is ultra delightful and fun. It's totally thrilling to have movement in your sex.

7 Have him thrust slowly and in longer movements, holding the in stroke for deeper, slower penetration. To switch it up, he can move the chair quickly and in shorter thrusts for more shallow penetration.

8 From the seated position, tilt your pelvis up, down, and in circles. This will access different hot spots for both of you.

♀ WHY IT WORKS FOR HER

★ You will be crazy for the clit stimulation in this move. And you will love the ease at which his penis moves in and out, giving longer and deeper penetration than ever before.

♂ WHY IT WORKS FOR HIM

★ Eye candy at it's best: this position gives him an amazing and unusual view of your pussy in motion, opening and closing. It really helps to have good pussy–eye coordination to make this position work, but once he gets it, he will love it.

RELATED MOVES

★ Supported on his knees, if the chair is wide enough, he can be on top.
Raise your pelvis upward.

★ From your seated position discussed above, put your feet on his chest. The weight of your feet feels good and is different than the usual hands. It can be sexy to have your feet on his chest. He can lick your toes.

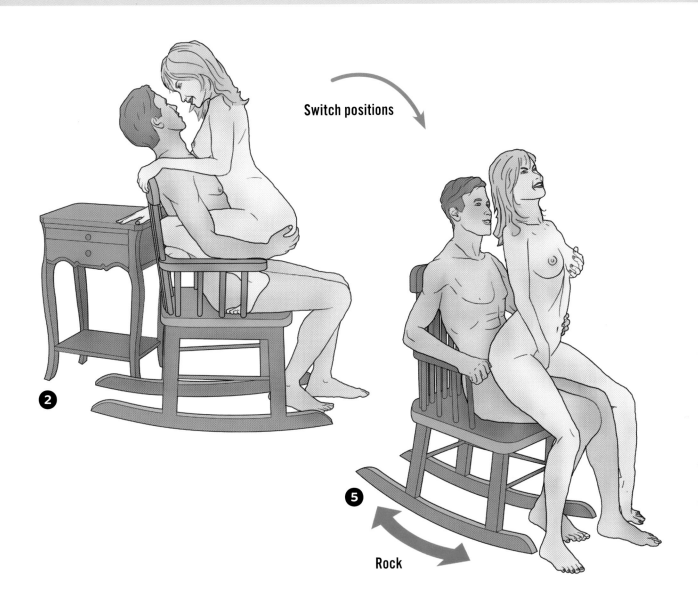

Switch positions

Rock

THE SEXPERT SAYS

How often have you left a sex session thinking that there was something off or not right about it? It could very well be that the thing that was off was your rhythm together. This position is perfect because rhythm is the focus. You will know quickly if you are not in time with each other. Take what you learned in the *Hard Rock* and bring the rhythm to your next sexual encounter.

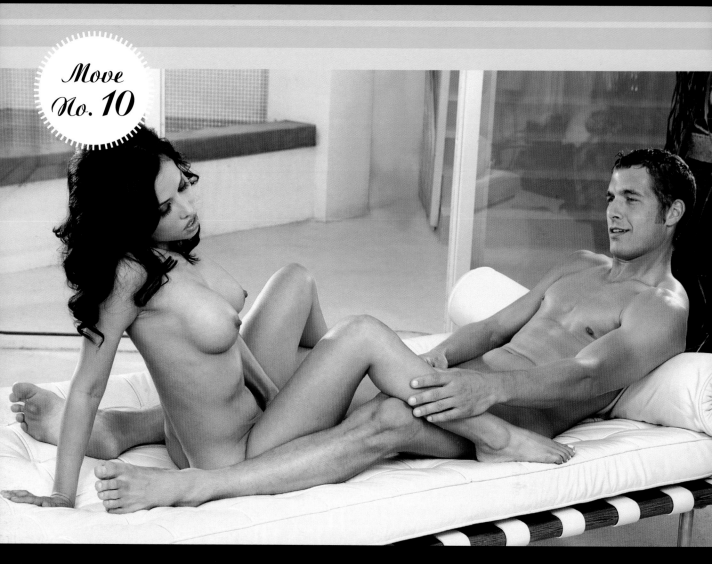

MUTUAL MASTURBATION PLAY-BY-PLAY

This is the ultimate crash course in how to please one another. Send your man to the moon and back, and let him watch as you ride your own cosmic wave. Reach orgasm describing the sexual play-by-play.

The Move: Mutual Masturbation Play-by-Play

THE PREPARATIONS

★ Think about your own sexual response cycle (SRC). Identify how you move through the cycle from early arousal to your refractory period. Pay attention to the following throughout your SRC:

— Fantasies

— Body postures

— Body movements

— Tensing of muscles

— Increased pulse

— Thoughts

— Feelings

— Rapid breathing

— Moans, groans, and other sounds

— Sex flush

★ As you masturbate, review your SRC and record the above items during each stage as closely as you can. For some stages, you may only have one or two items.

★ Pleasure yourself again, but this time say what you are thinking, feeling, and doing as you are doing it. This is practice for the actual move.

★ Turn on the heater. You will soon be naked with little body heat. Crank it up to a tropical 80°F (27°C).

★ Take off your clothes. Light candles or dim the lights. No darkness—you want your audience to be able to see this show.

THE LEAD-IN

Mutual masturbation is perfect for learning more about how your lover likes to be touched— and for those days that you are not feeling like having intercourse or oral sex but still want to orgasm.

Tell him that you would like to give him a play-by-play of your masturbation. Lead him to a comfortable place on the bed or floor.

THE FOREPLAY

① Sit facing each other, legs extended, so your left foot is at his right hip and your right foot is at his left hip.

THE SEXPERT SAYS

This move is actually a play-by-play guidebook or manual on how to be a great lover to one another. Think about it for a minute. You will witness and demonstrate the *exact* recipe for giving each other pleasure.

★ The Main Act

1. You can choose to keep your eyes open or closed. I suggest keeping your eyes closed so you can turn inward, narrating as you go along.

2. Get into position. Do you lie on your belly or your back?

3. Tell him what you are imagining or thinking. If cunnilingus is part of your fantasy, describe what you imagine his tongue, mouth, and hands are doing. Explain how you like to be licked and sucked from start to orgasm.

4. Touch yourself as you would if you were alone. Rub your clitoral hood, clitoral shaft, the urethra, the clitoral glans, the commisure, the labia minora, the anus.

5. Describe pressure, pace, rhythm, and direction in details: "I am using my index finger and doing a figure eight in the clockwise direction starting at the commisure and going down and around my clit. Mmm, that feels so good. Now, with my other hand, I am pinching my left nipple. Oh yeah, I'm closing the figure eight and going back over my vagina—it's oh-so wet—and up to the clitoris again, where I will run my finger left to right."

6. Reach for his hand and put it over yours so he can feel the pressure, pace, and rhythm of your motions.

7. Add sound. Moans and groans can be worth a thousand words. It's also okay to act out your fantasy instead of narrating it.

8. Use toys. Insert your dildo, explaining what you are doing: "I am inserting the dildo and pushing it toward my belly, imagining that it is your cock tapping my G-spot. Now I am going to point the dildo forward towards the end of my vagina."

9. Narrate the climax: "You touch my nipples with one hand and rub my clit with the other. That combination is making me come. I'm coming."

10. Don't forget the resolution: "I love to be held after I orgasm," as you snuggle up next to him.

♀ WHY IT WORKS FOR HER

★ This one move alone can save you hours of time and put you both on top of your game right away.

♂ WHY IT WORKS FOR HIM

★ This is a male fantasy come true: a hand that is not his own taking him on an orgasmic adventure that in his wildest, wettest dreams, he would never have guessed.

★ He gets the orgasm of his life and learns how to win with you every time. Men love to win, and they love to see their woman happy and sated.

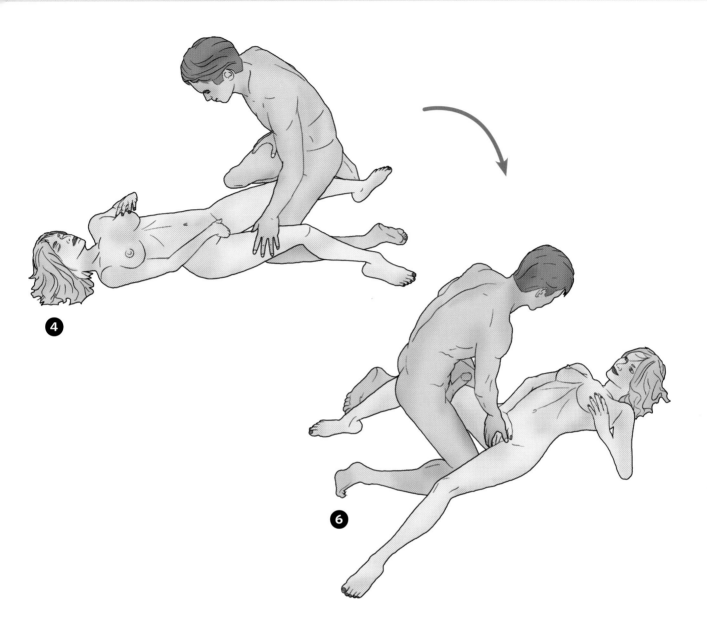

RELATED MOVES

★ Since you read this information, when he masturbates first ask him: "What are you doing now?" "Describe how it feels." "What are you thinking or imagining?" Ask this of him each time he shifts positions or techniques. When he is into rhythm, ask if you could put your hands over his. This is real hands-on training.

★ When he is all done, you will know everything from beginning to end, including thoughts of arousal, techniques, and what takes him over the top.

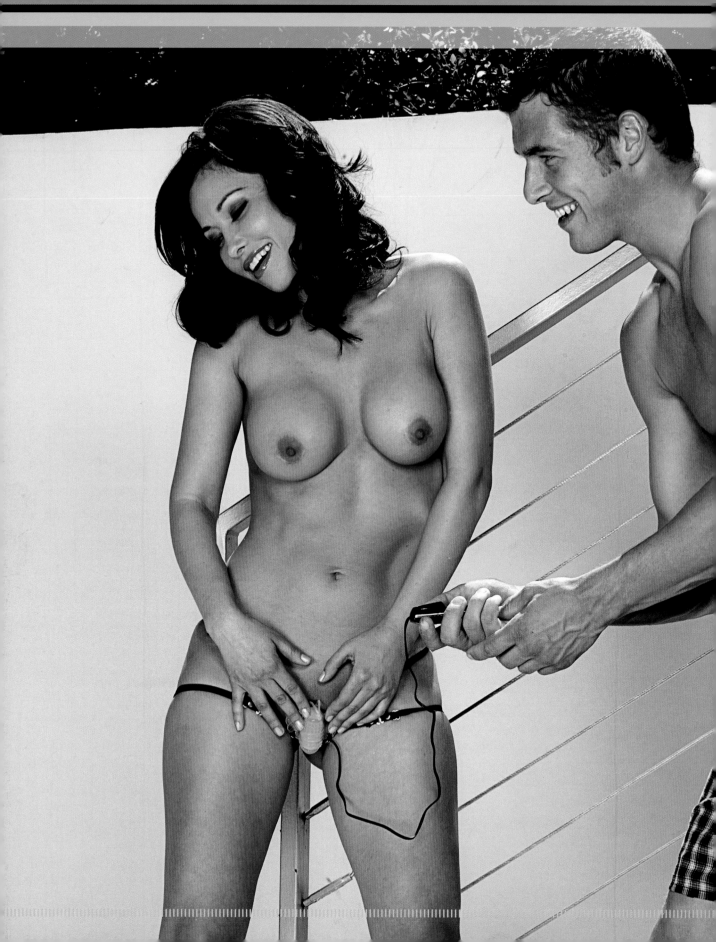

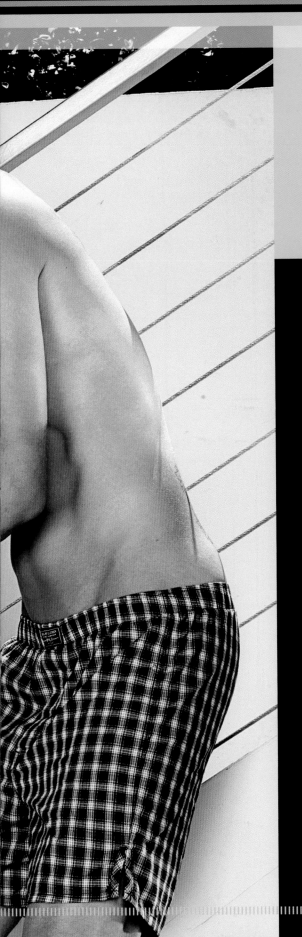

Standing

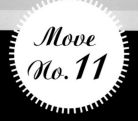

Move No. 11

DRESSED TO THRILL

Haven't you always wanted to rip off his shirt like a movie vixen? Give him an old shirt with loose buttons that will fly like confetti. Whip his ass with his own shirt (that's double naughty) and order him to rip off your clothes. Use the shirt as a sling around his hips to pull him into you.

The Move: Dressed to Thrill

THE PREPARATIONS

★ Pick out one of the button-down shirts that is in the giveaway pile.

★ Practice ripping off the shirt:

— One hand grabs the material on the left side between the buttons in the middles of the shirt and the other hand grabs the material on the right side.

— Hold on tight and in one swift move pull your hands in opposite directions.

★ If you can't find a shirt with buttons use a regular T-shirt:

— Using scissors, cut past the hem on the bottom or the collar at the top. This will give you a good start to the tear.

— Put one hand on the right and one on the left and in one swift movement, tear the shirt in half.

THE LEAD-IN

Put some life back into that old shirt by saying something like, "Hey, you are giving this shirt away? Let me see it on you first."

THE FOREPLAY

① When he puts that shirt on, really see him in it. What turns you on and makes you hot?

② Keep him in the shirt as you appreciate him. If he is trying to take it off, have him twirl around, show his muscles, or look in the mirror.

③ Feel your body filling up with sexual energy for him. Are you feeling aroused? Wet between the legs? Do you want to have sex with him at that moment? Did you have the image of him taking you from behind? Think of his perfect cock penetrating you.

④ When you have built up that sexual energy, walk toward him like a cat in heat. You need it. You want it.

||||||||||||||||||||||||||||||||||||||||||||||||||||||||||||||||||||||||||||||||||||||||||||||||||||||||||||

SEX FACT

An orgasm once or twice per week appears to strengthen the immune system's ability to resist flu and other viruses.

||||||||||||||||||||||||||||||||||||||||||||||||||||||||||||||||||||||||||||||||||||||||||||||||||||||||||||

THE SEXPERT SAYS

As with any of the other moves where you are both getting out of your comfort zone and trying something new, there is an opportunity here to create safety. The other person might be feeling a little vulnerable or maybe even silly at moments. Celebrating each other will create a safety that will inspire hotter, more creative sex in the future.

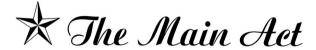 # The Main Act

1 Take a breath of courage and talk dirty, getting as nasty as you can get.

2 Put your hands on the shirt—along the buttons in the button-down or the tear spot of the T-shirt—and rip it off in one swift swoop, like during a Brazilian wax or ripping off a Band-Aid.

3 Throw the shirt aside and rub your naked chests together immediately.

4 Remove the rest of your own and his clothes with almost as much enthusiasm, but keeping the stitching.

5 From the standing position, wrap the shirt around his waist and pull him to you and inside of you. Go right to the act of penetration like a pair of wild animals, ravishing each other, letting his passion fuel your own and vice versa until you are a big ball of hot monkey love.

6 Bend over and beg for him to give it to you doggy style as you howl in delight. Allow the calls of the wild to come out of your mouth without a filter. Creating the space for this to happen will give his wild beast permission to do the same.

7 Animals in the wild don't care about giving each other pleasure. Go for your own here (with love, of course), growling, howling, huffing, and puffing until you both collapse in orgasmic relief.

♀ WHY IT WORKS FOR HER

★ She experiences the exhilaration and freedom of going wild.

♂ WHY IT WORKS FOR HIM

★ Men fantasize about ripping off your clothes and having their clothes ripped off in the passion of the moment. For some, it is the ultimate expression of "I want you. I desire you. Take me now."

RELATED MOVES

★ Choose a button-down and tell him to rip off your shirt.

★ Receive him by ripping off your own shirt.

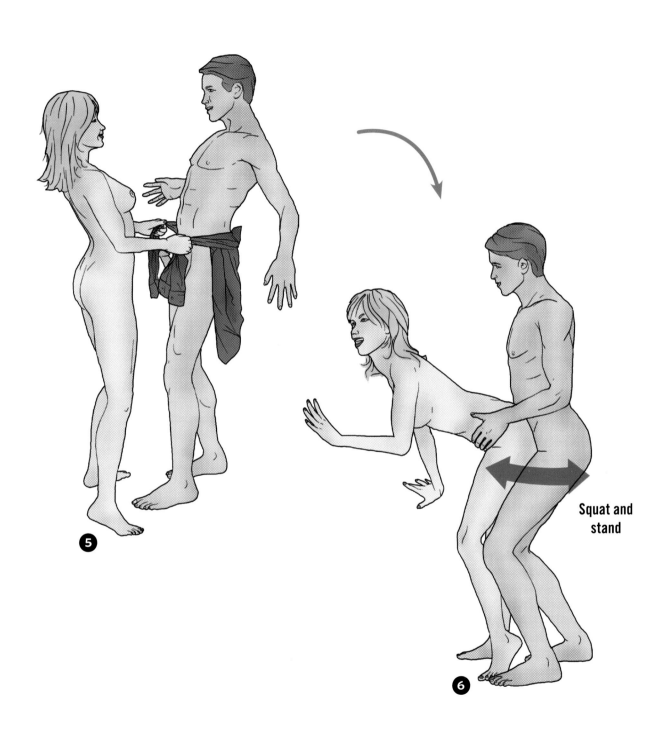

Squat and
stand

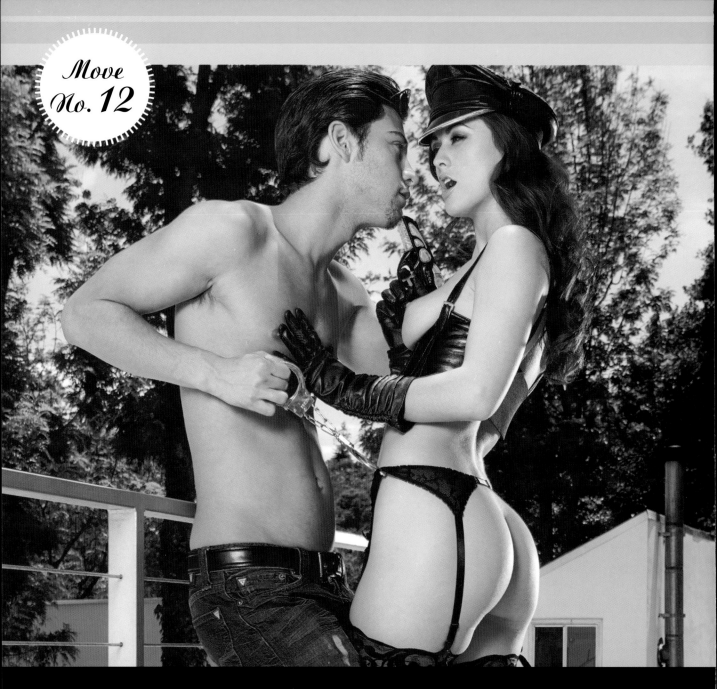

UP AGAINST THE WALL

Load your water pistols and play cop. Whoever is in charge orders the other against the
wall, hands up. He may tell you to face the wall and spread your legs wide, angling your ass
out to him. Or you may tell him to use the wall as a brace when you mount him, with one
leg wrapped around his waist.

The Move: Up Against the Wall

THE PREPARATIONS

★ Load your water pistols. Handcuffs optional.

★ If you are not practiced in directing, try watching yourself in the mirror while giving sexy orders. Keep working on your dialogue until you are able to become aroused when giving orders.

THE LEAD-IN

Give him a "citation" for peeing on the toilet, leaving the cap off the toothpaste, or something not too serious.

When he demands to know what that is all about, pull out your "failure to appear and clean up your mess" notice. Show him the water pistol in your other hand.

Walk him up to the wall (you big bully) and order him to put his arms up, back to the wall, and spread his legs.

Do a pat-down search stopping at his package. "What is this?"

Pull down his pants and order him *not* to get an erection as you put your mouth to his cock.

THE FOREPLAY

① Slide your gun up his inner thighs and around his balls, while reminding him that "around these parts, we leave the toilet seat down."

② Put the water pistol in between his cheeks and pull the trigger. Woohoo! This may or may not qualify as foreplay depending on the man. It will definitely be refreshing and maybe even funny.

③ If he puts up a struggle—or even if he doesn't—cuff his hands behind his back as you have your way teasing his cock in your mouth.

SEX FACTS

• According to the MSNBC/*Elle* survey, 34 percent of respondents have talked about or acted out sexual fantasies to spice up their sex life in the last year.

• The *Cosmopolitan*/Durex survey found that 33.5 percent of respondents have thought about another man (or a cop) while having sex with their partner.

⭐ The Main Act

① Stand closely, face to face, bodies pressed together, with his back against the wall.

② In a calm but authoritative voice, whisper in his ear to bend his knees slightly so he will be in alignment to enter you.

③ If you want to take the cuffs off, make a deal with him that if you uncuff him, he needs to follow orders closely.

④ If the cuffs are still on, make sure he is standing against the wall and you are holding on to him for balance of both of you.

⑤ Stand in front of him and tell him to straighten his legs and insert his penis into your vagina.

⑥ Now he can squat and stand for repetitive penetration in and out, in and out.

⑦ When the time is right, tell him that you are a naughty cop and he needs to serve justice using his cock and the handcuffs.

♀ WHY IT WORKS FOR HER

★ Changing energies from masculine to feminine or dominant to submissive is fun and empowering, and can be a great learning tool, especially if you have a tendency to play out one more than the other.

♂ WHY IT WORKS FOR HIM

★ Being submissive allows him to relax and let you take control for a change.

RELATED MOVES

★ Do a good ole Western draw. Whoever gets squirted with water first gets to choose to be the naughty cop or bad guy or gal.

THE SEXPERT SAYS

We all experience moments when we would like ourselves or our lovers to be more dominant or more submissive. But generally speaking, men report that their erections seem to come out of nowhere when they are giving orders to their lovers. Good to know when someone wants to summon up an erection.

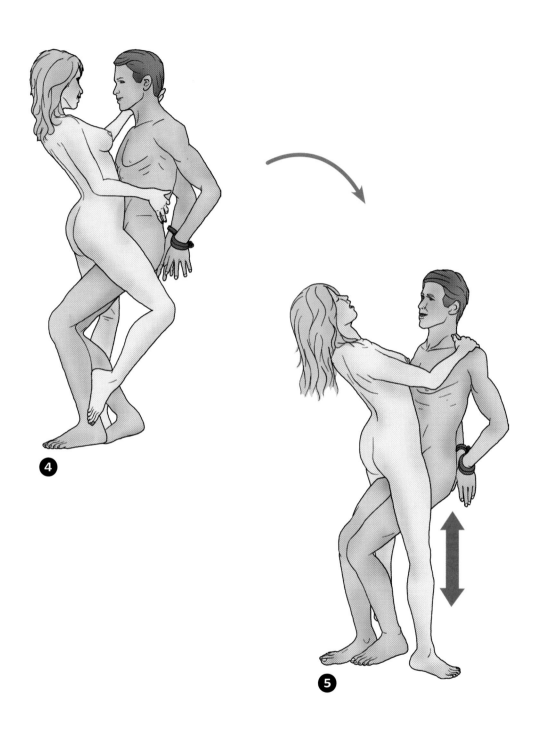

4

5

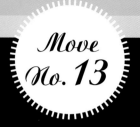

Move No. 13

QUIET RIOT

Show your appreciation for that rock concert. Unzip/unbutton his pants, take his drink, raise your skirt, and give him your leg to hold while he gives you his quiet riot in the standing-room-only concert.

The Move: Quiet Riot

THE PREPARATIONS

★ Plant the sex-in-public seed a few days prior, by saying something like, "I'd love to have that public quickie we talked about." He may be really excited about the idea but not the act. Ask him and find out if there is a difference.

★ If you want a chance to dress sexy, maybe even a little trashy, a rock concert might be it. Choose a loose flowing skirt and no panties, for easy access of course. This position is standing, so if he is taller than you, choose heels. If he is equal in height or shorter, go for the flats. The rest is up to you.

★ Begin the fun before the concert by putting a little female arousal cream on your clit while you're getting dressed. This is an amazing little secret. Every day is a great day with this stuff.

★ Pack your remote-control wireless panty vibe. Concerts are the best place for these noisy little buggers.

★ A public quickie requires some groundwork in the form of heavy flirting. Investing your time up front in foreplay will make up for less real-time penetration.

★ When you are driving in the car on the way to the concert, flirt.

★ When you catch him staring at your radiance, I dare you to stare back at him and hold it. All too often, we get uncomfortable and look away. Once you get his attention, look at him with an "I want you" look. If you have trouble mustering up a look, imagine sexy scenes with him and the "I want you" look will naturally emerge.

★ Once you have his attention, direct it to your best assets by touching your breasts, your ass, or your neck; running your fingers through your hair; sticking out your breasts; or flashing him your starlight smile.

★ If he is shy, make the first move and ask him if he likes what you are wearing as you run his hand up the inside of your thighs and to the wireless vibrating bullet.

★ Turn on the vibrator, letting him hear and see you become aroused. Tell him that you will give him control when you get to the concert.

THE LEAD-IN

Hand him the remote, turn around, and smile as you head down to the concert floor. If he doesn't follow, take him by the hand and lead him to an open space where you can let him see you dancing and enjoying the vibrations.

THE FOREPLAY

① Find the beat of a slow song as you sway and swagger your hips back and forth, round and round, slowly and sensually. Roll your shoulders toward him and away. Run your hands through your hair, exposing your neck. Raise your arms, close your eyes, and feel the music. Turn around and give him a view. Occasionally, move in close enough so he can feel the warmth of your breath on his neck and your perky nipples brushing up against his chest. Step back again so he can watch some more and continue enjoying the tease.

② Ultimately, move in close to him so your bodies are touching. Wrap your hands around his neck so you are feeling the back of his head.

||||||||||||||||||||||||||||||||||||||||||||||||||||||||||||||||||||||||||||||||||||||||||||||||||||||||||||||||||||||||||||||

THE SEXPERT SAYS

Flirting can be in the form of conversation, body language, or physical contact. Do women know how to flirt or even reciprocate a flirt? Men approach us, and all we have to do is decide yes or no. The problem with that? We attract attention from every man in the room, including those we don't care to notice. If passively waiting to be chosen, hopefully by someone you like, has been your approach, it's time to change your game and have more fun by being an active flirt.

★ The Main Act

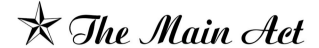

1 While your bodies are touching in a close embrace, lift your skirt so it is up in the front and draped down on the sides and in the back.

2 Undo his pants, reach in, take out his cock, and put it inside of you.

3 Lift up one leg and put it on his waist for him to hold on to. Look into each other's eyes, not at his penis or what is going on below the waist.

4 Push into each other with a slow, sensual, bump and grind, feeling the vibration of the music as you both come to climax.

> *Disclaimer: Public play can be exciting and highly erotic, but there can be legal ramifications, so be discreet.*

♀ WHY IT WORKS FOR HER

★ The close body contact and rubbing up and down gives added stimulation to the clitoris. There is a lot of flirting in here, which is an excellent practice for any woman who wants to learn how to seduce these easy but lovely creatures.

♂ WHY IT WORKS FOR HIM

★ This position is a sexy, confident, sexual move that makes a man feel sexually attractive and more wanted than anyone in the room. It sends the message that she wants him now and doesn't want to wait. Most men don't want to wait. They fantasize about having sex with their lover while everyone else is going about their business.

RELATED MOVES

★ Raise and lower yourself on your toes for deeper penetration and lustier thrusting.

SEX FACT

According to an ABC News Live Poll, 57 percent of Americans have had sex in public.

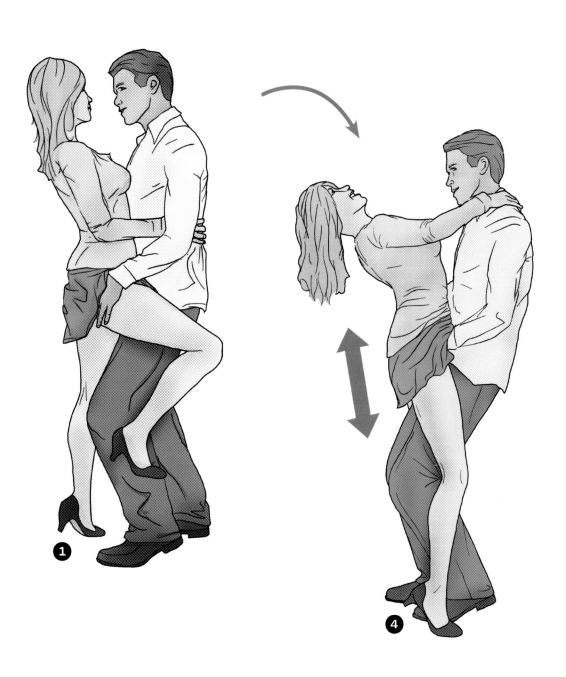

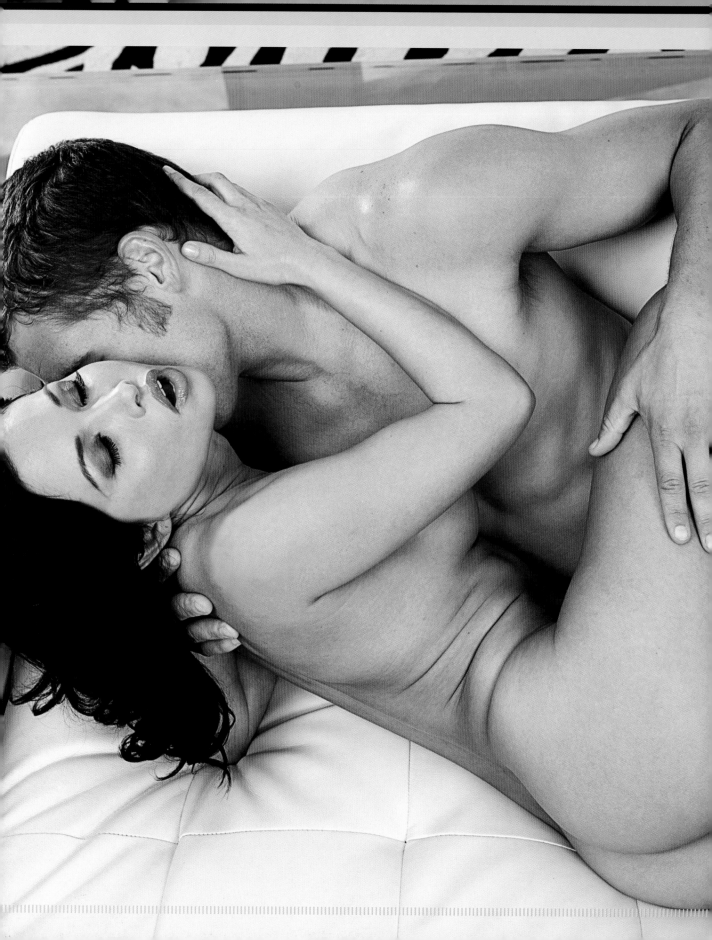

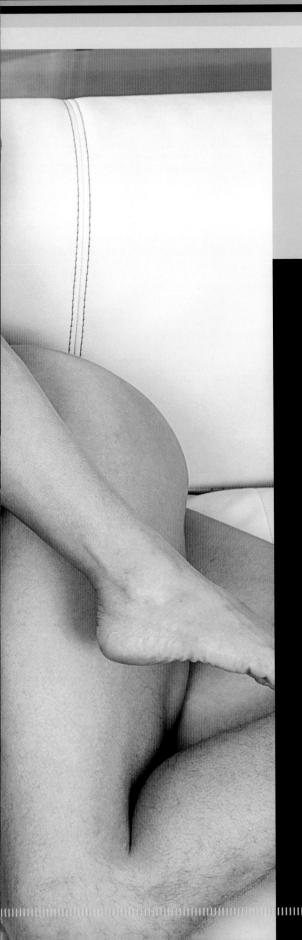

Side by Side

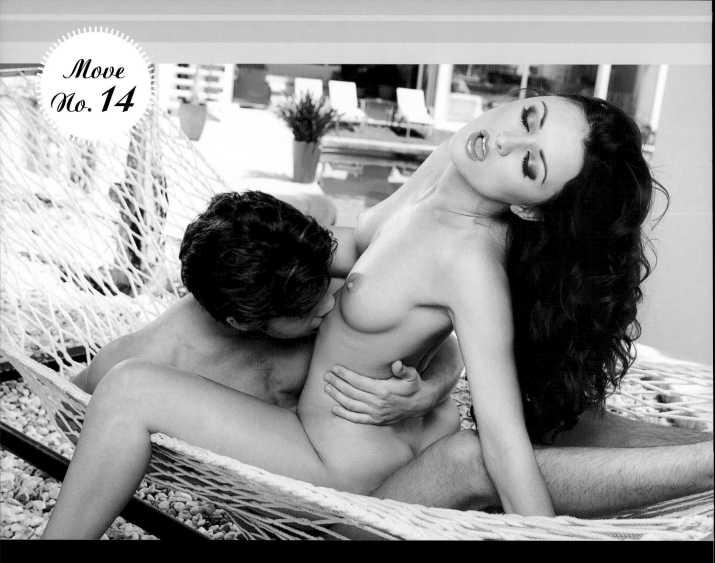

CLOUD 9

On a lazy summer day, lead him to the hammock, where he can lie on his back and contemplate the sky. After a brief respite of cloud watching, join him naked in the hammock and envelope yourselves in this lovely side-by-side position as you are suspended from the trees.

The Move: Cloud 9

THE PREPARATIONS

★ Don't have a hammock? Get one. There are hammocks that you can suspend in your backyard between trees or in your home from a hammock stand.

★ After you hang the hammock, get some practice and learn how to move and shift in your new, suspended sex platform. Part of the thrill of this position is the sensation that you just might tip over onto the floor.

★ Red heels are a great visual, but this position is a jaw-dropper with or without them.

★ Grab your cell phone. You are going to call him.

★ Play some music that makes you feel sexy.

THE LEAD-IN

Get naked and lie in the hammock. Let the netting pattern your beautiful naked skin. Arrange the netting so your nipples protrude through the net. Always too shy to wear fishnet stockings? Girl, look at you now!

Call him on his cell.

When he comes into sight, extend your bare leg out like a flag. Instant erection for him.

When he notices your nipples, glide your finger over them.

THE FOREPLAY

① Hang your legs over the hammock, opening yourself up. Tease and titillate him with your net show.

② Move your legs to the music, pointing your toes and pedaling your imaginary bike with slow sensuality. Open them spread-eagle as you yearn for his touch. Cross them like scissors and open them up for a window of opportunity to enter or just look inside. Lock them shut. He's missed his chance. Maybe you'll open them again for him soon.

③ Cover your vulva with the netting. Take his hand and slip one of his fingers through the net and into your pussy.

④ He is standing facing you and you are sitting in the hammock, legs spread, with feet on the floor, the hammock holding most of your weight.

⑤ Instruct him to push the hammock up and position himself between your legs so he can enter you.

⑥ Tilt your pelvis up to the clouds. From here you can raise one or both legs, putting them to his chest. In this position he has direct access to your G-spot. What a nice way to start.

⭐ *The Main Act*

1 Carefully get into the sideways position. If you try to roll into the sideways position on the hammock, you will likely roll right off, which would be funny but not part of the move per se. Grab his ass, pulling him in close to you.

2 He is in the perfect place for some ass play. Separate those cheeks, and knead and push them into you to really prime the pump.

3 Put your feet in between the netting for leveraging power.

4 Tilt your pelvis forward and backward to access all the right spots, finding the spot that feels really good to you.

5 While having intercourse, insert your hand into the perfect amount space between your bodies for stroking his balls and your clitoris. Most women cannot climax without some sort of clitoral stimulation. If he doesn't naturally go for the clit, go for it yourself, rubbing and thrusting to an off-the-charts orgasm.

♀ WHY IT WORKS FOR HER

★ The fresh air and the sun on your skin is enough to make this a good day. Throw in vaginal penetration and clitoral stimulation and this is like being on cloud 9.

♂ WHY IT WORKS FOR HIM

★ Seeing your sexiness all wrapped up in the netting and it making patterns on your skin will have him seriously thinking he is on cloud 9.

★ Gravity is his friend during the foreplay position, allowing for deep penetration without the work.

RELATED MOVE

★ Flip onto your stomach for rear-entry penetration and access to your G-spot. The potential to tip out of the hammock is an arousing thought that will keep him on his toes.

THE SEXPERT SAYS

It's not too hot for sex; it's time for hotter sex. Sex and sun go great together. Libidos rise when we're outside feeling energized and healthy.

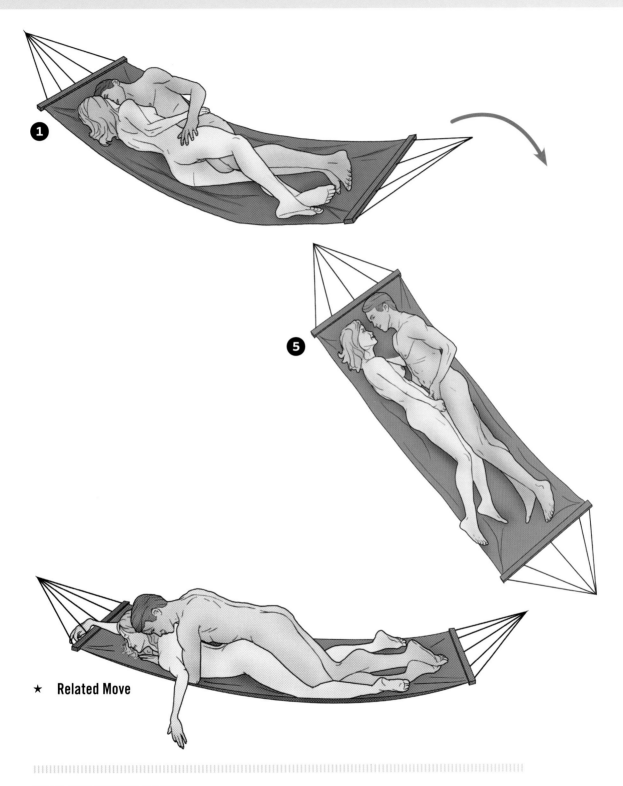

★ **Related Move**

THE SEXPERT SAYS

Askmen.com has rated being in nature as one of the "top 5 must-try outdoor sex experiences."

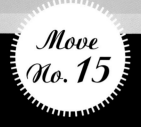

Move No. 15

THE UGLY CHAIR

You have asked him, begged him, pleaded with him to get rid of that ugly reclining chair. Stop hating the furniture. Turn that recliner into a beautiful sex throne for a sideways position.

The Move: The Ugly Chair

THE PREPARATIONS

★ Clean the ugly chair or cover it with your favorite fabric. He won't care either way once his cock is in your mouth. The most important thing is that you are able to lounge in that chair with comfort. If it is a reclining chair, put the footrest down and his arms to the side.

★ Put on something that makes you feel sexy.

THE LEAD-IN

He probably watches evening TV from the ugly chair, which means you know when you can strike.

Walk toward him slowly while making eye contact. When you get to the chair, moving your pelvis in hip rolls, raise your arms and run your fingers through your hair.

Place your hands on the back of the chair so you can lean in and show him your breasts.

Raise your leg to the chair and show off. Touch your body and feel good.

Put one hand on the chair and rub the side of your body up and down his crotch.

THE FOREPLAY

① Now is the time for some contact.

② Do pelvic thrusts on his leg and his crotch. Move to the side, the left or right, so you are horizontal on his lap and can show off your sexy curves and your butt.

③ Do the butt grind. Turn your head so you are looking at him and roll your butt in front of him. Put your right or left leg on the chair, touching your butt and leg. Touch your hair, spank yourself, lift up your skirt. Sit down on his pelvic area and lightly roll up and down on his crotch. Lean your body onto him and touch his head. Open your shirt and give him a peak. Can he hold your leg up so he can see more curves?

④ Slowly remove your bottoms and his.

||||||||||||||||||||||||||||||||||||||||||||||||||||||||||||||||||||||||||||||||||||||||||||||||||||||||||||||||||||||

SEX FACTS

• According to the AOL Health and *Glamour* Men's Sex Survey, 24 percent of men have reported that they have faked an orgasm during intercourse. (Yes, it does happen!) On the other hand, the ABC News American Sex Survey found that 48 percent of women have faked an orgasm. (Probably in a hurry to get out of the ugly chair!)

• According to the *Cosmopolitan*/Durex survey, 62 percent of respondents reported that they sometimes climax at the same time.

||||||||||||||||||||||||||||||||||||||||||||||||||||||||||||||||||||||||||||||||||||||||||||||||||||||||||||||||||||||

THE SEXPERT SAYS

Don't hesitate going for your own pleasure during sex. Partners who climax together usually report it is because they are brought over the top from hearing and seeing their partners approach orgasm. Men will catch your wave, but for him to do that, you have to *authentically allow* yourself to experience and express pleasure. Let me explain how this works: an experienced man will know a woman's sexual response cycle either consciously from reading or subconsciously from observing other women or knowing his own cycles, since they are much the same. A man will get aroused not because he likes the timbre of your moan, but because it signifies arousal and pleasure that he is a part of.

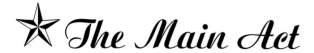

★ The Main Act

1 Recline the ugly chair and lie down facing each other.

2 The ugly chair is perfect for sex because it never fully reclines. There is always a gap where you can place your leg so it doesn't get squished. Have him pull you close and penetrate you.

3 Put one foot on the footrest and use that for leverage to move yourself up and down. You can also put the other leg behind him against the armrest so you can have better control and range of movement.

♀ WHY IT WORKS FOR HER

★ The face-to-face, toe-to-toe position is very intimate, and the gap created by the reclining chair helps make space for either you or him to access your clitoris and nipples.

★ Everything is energy. If sex in the easy chair is not the equivalent of flowers and candle-light, allow his reaction to be your arousal. Allow his joy to be what gets you wet between the legs. Leading this move is not only a playful act, but also is a statement that you are in control of your happiness—you choose to be happy, and that is very, very sexy.

♂ WHY IT WORKS FOR HIM

★ The gap allows for you to reach around and pull his butt to you. Seems simple, but even the slightest gesture of this nature registers in a man's mind as "she really wants me."

★ Sex in the ugly chair is right up there with sex in his car and swallowing his semen: you are accepting him and the things that make him happy.

RELATED MOVES

★ The woman-on-top position is really great here. Again, this gap when the chair is reclined is a blessing, making for a little lift in his butt. You can also put a pillow down so he can rest into it.

THE SEXPERT SAYS

Every woman needs to feel the power that she has, and *you do* have power. Here is a secret that few women know: he knows that you know you have the power, and he loves that fact. He loves surrendering to your seduction and witnessing a woman in her sexual power.

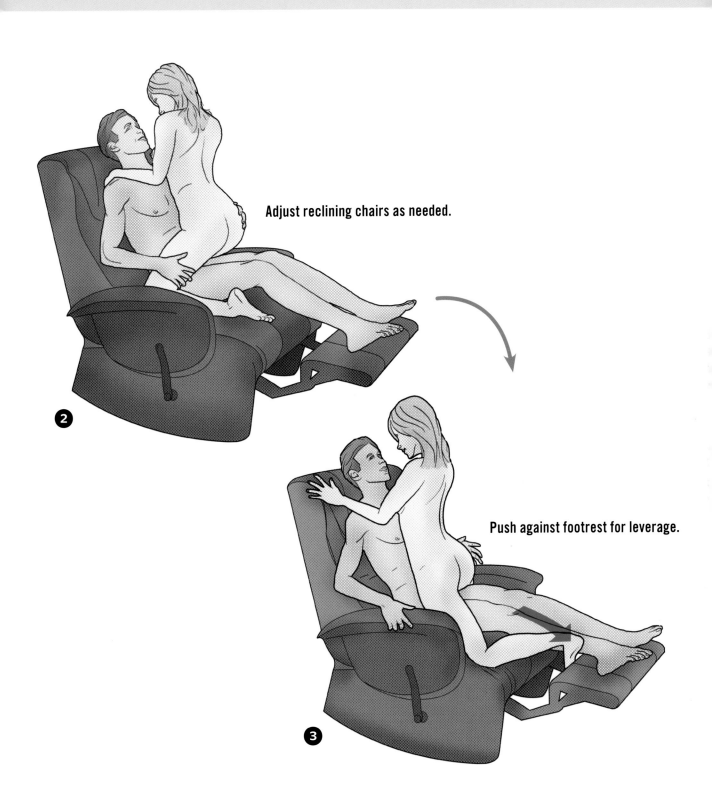

Adjust reclining chairs as needed.

❷

Push against footrest for leverage.

❸

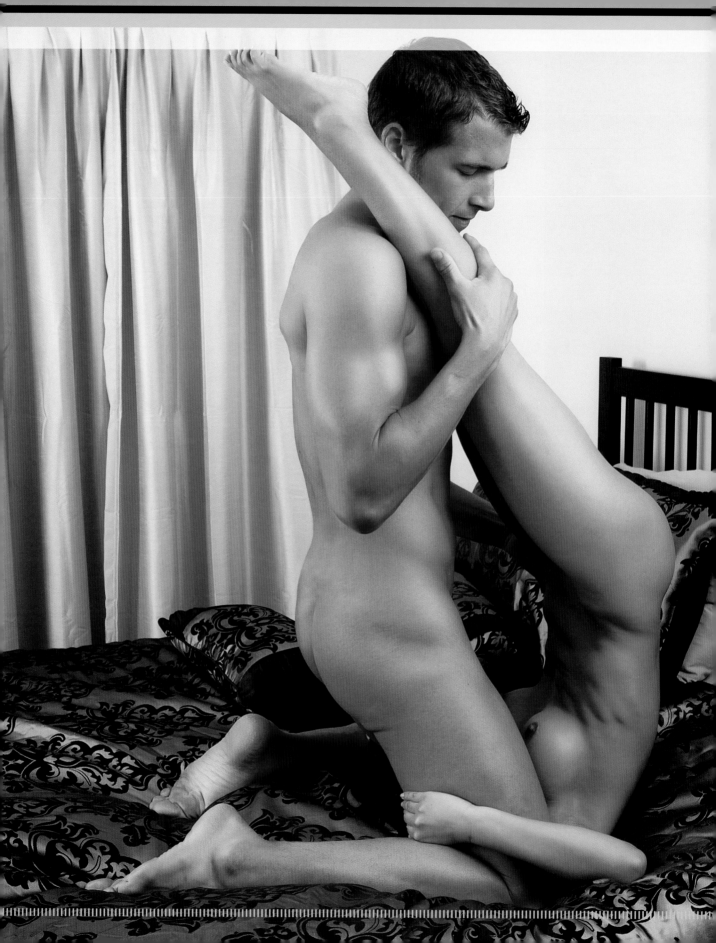

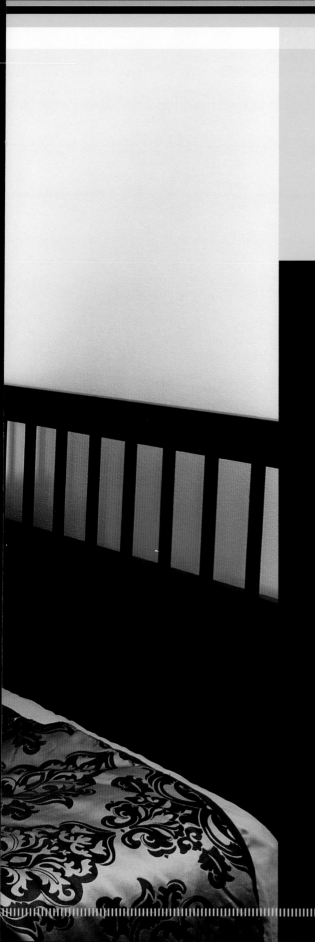

Blow Jobs

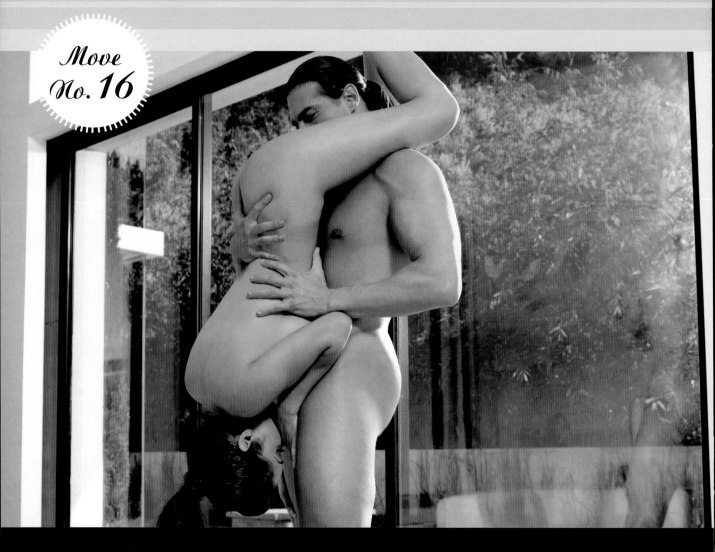

FOR THE LOVE OF HONEY

The Move: For the Love of Honey

THE PREPARATIONS

★ Vacuum the surrounding area in the bedroom and dust in all those places you don't normally see. You don't want to have to be looking at dust bunnies while giving this inverted blow job. It can be too distracting, and even if it is a subconscious thought, it will take away from the power of the BJ.

★ Practice getting in the position for a few days, holding the position for a little more time (seconds) each day. Being slightly inverted is not something we are used to. A gradual build will help you relax into the position and have fun.

★ Have a mutual masturbation session with him. While you are stroking yourselves, go through the sexual response cycle, sharing where you are on a scale from 1 to 10. Identify 1 as being early arousal, 10 as being resolution, and everything else as in between. After you climax together and are in the post-orgasm snuggle, debrief the 1 to 10 scale by sharing your thoughts and techniques.

THE LEAD-IN

Get into a lip-lock, making out all the way to the bed. When you get to the edge of the bed, move your oral attentions down to his pants.

Look up at him and ask him if he wants to go real deep in your mouth, so deep that he will feel the back of your throat with the tip of his cock. Chances are good you will get a yes.

THE FOREPLAY

① Foreplay is very, very important. After all, how long can you be upside down for?

② Do what you did in the mutual masturbation exercise a day prior, only this time, you are doing it to him. If he had a threesome fantasy at 1 and was giving himself a five-finger slow stroke to his cock, retell the fantasy and give the same moves (or as close as possible). Don't worry about being perfect. Have him yell out the number as you progress. When you get to 8, move to the headstand position.

THE SEXPERT SAYS

No one says you have to swallow or deep throat. But if that is something you can do, men love it! They often report that taking him in deep lets him know that you want him deeply. Swallowing his spunk is accepting him.

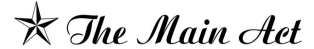

The Main Act

1 Have him spot you, while you do a headstand on the mattress. In the position, you should be looking at his cock upside down. Have him kneel down so his cock can enter your mouth.

2 Put one hand between your mouth and his cock, allowing him to thrust at a comfortable pace for you. And put one hand on his pelvic bone so you can guide him in the thrusting into your mouth.

3 Use your hands to create a slow, steady build. The penis becomes desensitized just like the clitoris. Too much too soon can make for a long session.

4 If he starts becoming all crazy and fucking your face, which could happen, place a relatively firm grip on the base of his cock, so he can feel the tightness of your hand that your lips could provide in an otherwise short rendezvous.

5 Cup his balls, or whatever move you do to bring him to orgasm quickly.

♀ WHY IT WORKS FOR HER

★ The beauty of this position is that you are bypassing the gag reflex as he goes deep, all the way to the back of your throat. The ejaculate will shoot to the back of your throat, allowing you to swallow without tasting.

★ You are giving him a tremendous gift and also waving a red flag that says you are playful, sexy, and up for new things.

♂ WHY IT WORKS FOR HIM

★ First of all, any woman who is willing to go upside down to give him an amazing oral experience is freaking hot and a keeper.

★ He will love this position because he has the feeling of control, even though you and I both know you are controlling the depth and pace.

★ He will get to go deep and reach the caverns of your throat—and ejaculate in your mouth.

RELATED MOVES

★ If you are feeling like you are going to gag, push the back of your tongue to the roof of your mouth, creating an artificial back of the throat that he can tap with his penis.

★ When he pulls out, offer suction and purse your lips closed.

SEX FACT

According to an Askmen.com sex survey, 25 percent of men rate oral sex as their favorite sex act.

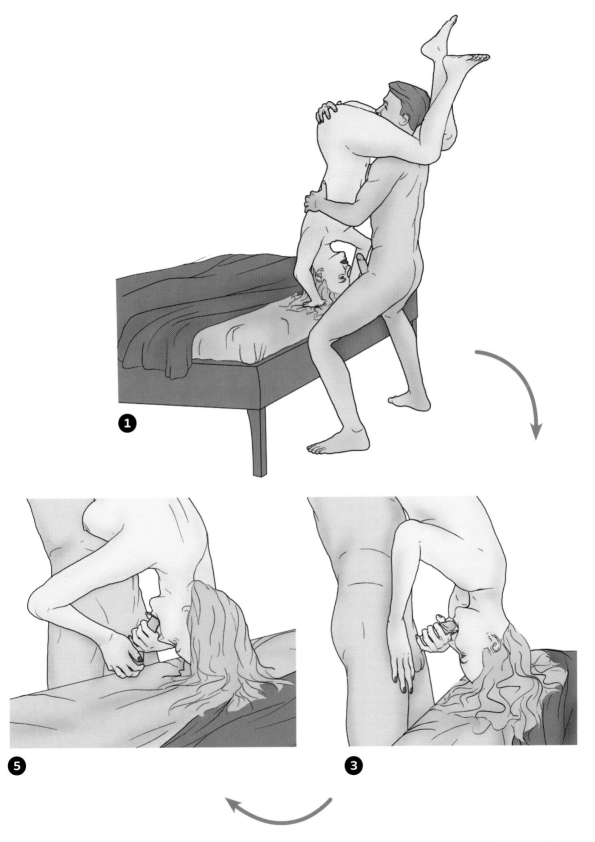

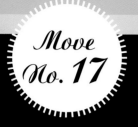

Move
No. 17

THE HEARTBEAT BJ

Take his hand in yours and hold your lips to his wrist until you feel his heartbeat in your lips. Kiss him slowly all down his body. As you perform the BJ, keep one hand on his heart.

The Move: The Heartbeat BJ

THE PREPARATIONS

★ The power of a BJ is in the intention. Spend some time getting clear on what that is: what do you love, like, or appreciate about the man or the moment?

★ Set the mood with candles, music, and a no-clutter space.

THE LEAD-IN

Hold eye contact for a few moments and send your intention to him through your eyes. Speak softly or whisper in his ear what you want to do to him.

Synchronize your breathing.

Put your head on his heart and your hand on the pulse in his wrist, listening and feeling him. Think of the beat of his heart as if it were a musical beat. If the beat were a song, would it be a ballad, jazz, classical, metal, new age? Feel his song.

THE FOREPLAY

① Move your body across his in time with the beat of his heart. Glide your lips across his neck and ears, breathing warmth on to his skin.

② Put your arms on his shoulders and lean your pelvis in to rub your vulva against his cock. Enjoy the rubbing sensations on your clit for a moment.

③ Let your desire dictate the pressure, speed, and intensity of your movements. When you feel the erotic charge, send it back to him in the form of a moan.

④ Keep one hand on his heart as you listen to his breath. Hear what his body has to say. Feel the beat in your pussy.

⑤ Remember your intention as you make your way down his body and put your mouth around his beautiful cock. Count the ways you love his penis and get ready to orally express yourself.

⑥ Allow the beat of his heart to be the base for your dance and inspire your moves in this epic blow job.

SEX FACTS

• At orgasm, the heart averages 140 beats per minute for men and women.

• Studies have shown that men who have at least three orgasms per week are 50 percent less likely to die of heart disease.

THE SEXPERT SAYS

Much of our lovemaking is not about what we can see, but rather what we can feel. We can be most successful at connecting in lovemaking if we can learn to read each other's energy in an instant. To start, try this exercise: Blindfold yourself. In an open space, have him move slowly and without words around the room as you follow his energy. Switch. Notice how much of your exchange is felt, how much of it is a knowing, a feeling. Read your lover's energy and adapt your lovemaking accordingly.

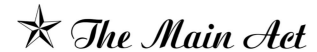

The Main Act

1 Run your nose and lips around his balls and his pubic area. Follow the trail of your nose and lips with the fingers of your free hand as you glide to his inner thighs and between his ass cheeks.

2 Starting at the base, move your mouth up and over the head of his cock and down the side of the shaft as if it were a harmonica. Cover every inch of skin while humming your favorite ditty. Repeat.

3 Add suction and release saliva.

4 Starting at the tip of his head, suck all the way down to the base. This move is called "Sucking the Mango Fruit." Repeat several times.

5 When you have taken him in as far as you can, press the back of your tongue to the roof of your mouth. This is the "French Press." Match the press to the beating of his heart. Remember, listen for his heartbeat. Move in time with his heart, as if you were a musician in a jam session.

6 From the French Press, drop some saliva down his cock and put the pointer finger and thumb of your free hand together to form an "A-okay" gesture. Place the A-okay under your lips and grip the penis lightly but firmly, increasing the intensity of sensation.

7 Move your mouth up and down in time to the song of his heart and allow your hand to follow behind. Add suction and tongue to the head and pressure with your hands as you bring him to orgasm.

♀ WHY IT WORKS FOR HER

★ This move provides a really sensual and sexy way to connect.

♂ WHY IT WORKS FOR HIM

★ A BJ with beat, the Heartbeat BJ will have him feeling a connection to you that he may or may not be able to explain.

RELATED MOVES

★ Gently squeeze his penis in a loose grip. Move up and down, to the beat of his heart.

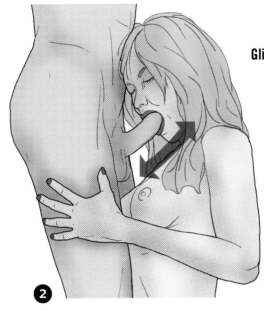

Glide mouth over the head
and along the side.

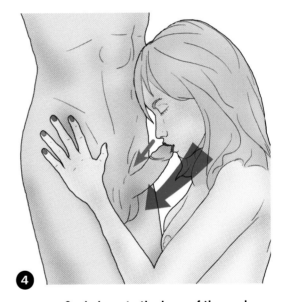

Suck down to the base of the cock.

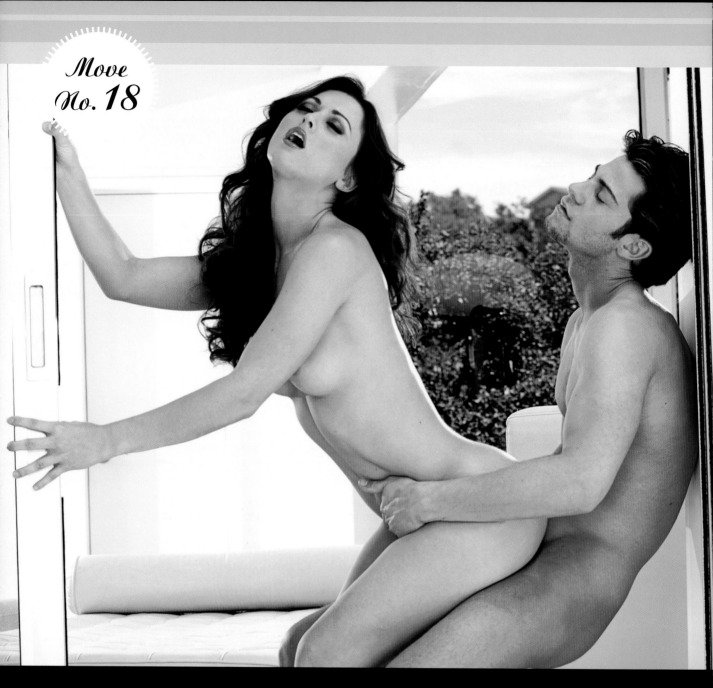

THE DOOR JAM

Get your man's guns in shape and give him a blow job at the same time. As he's using a pull-up bar setup between the doorjambs, you take care of his cock. He does a pull-up and wraps his legs around your neck, giving you easy access.

The Move: The Door Jam

THE PREPARATIONS

★ If you don't already have one, put up an exercise bar on your bedroom door. At a fraction of the cost of a gym membership, he can shape up while you give him much more fun.

★ Attempt these exercises before making him work for his BJ. Most people, whether they are men or women, find pull-ups to be a challenge.

Pull-Up

★ Grab the bar with palms facing away from you and shoulder-width apart. Pull up all the way, slowly, until your chin passes the bar. This exercise works the muscles of the back, biceps, and forearms.

★ If he cannot do any pull-ups, try negatives. Negatives are half pull-ups. Place a chair or stool under his feet or assist him by lifting him up as you fellate him.

★ If negatives don't work, start with a flexed arm hang. It's still hot to see him hanging there, arms extended and completely vulnerable.

Wide-Grip Pull-Up

★ Take an overhand grip on a high horizontal bar with your hands placed 7 to 10 inches (18 to 25 cm) wider than your shoulders, or about two hands away from a chin-up. Inhale slightly and raise your shoulders first while holding your elbows out to your sides and concentrating on pulling your elbows down to raise your body. Continue to pull yourself up until your chin is level with or slightly above the bar. This exercise is great for developing mass in the upper latissimus dorsi, but it's a tough one. You can do partial reps, which are just as effective by simply raising and lowering your shoulders.

THE LEAD-IN

If you can't do some sort of "up," simply hang from the bar and reel him in with your legs by opening them up, grabbing him, and pulling him into you. When you capture him, bring him toward you and tell him how hot it would be if he sucked on your breasts and fingered you while in the wide-open position.

THE FOREPLAY

① After he fulfills your request, have him get on the bar. When he is in the midst of his pull-up, gently run your fingers over his package. Unless he has the focus of Superman and can shoot red lasers from his eyes, he will likely laugh at your playful suggestion.

② Tell him to hold on while you pull out his penis. Remember, there are different types of pull-ups; choose the one that is most fitting for him. You want him to be a success and blow him.

③ Pull-ups are supposed to be slow and mindful. Most people move up and down way too quickly, trying to just get through them.

★ The Main Act

1 Time to help him work those guns! Tell him that if he wants the full BJ he must earn it and listen to his master, I mean coach.

2 Start with a simple arm extension. Lube your hand and stroke his cock from bottom to top and over the head with a loose grip. Let him go and give him a little playful swing.

3 Give him a little push so his body is swinging. Using no hands, try to catch his penis in your mouth as it comes toward you. Put a hand on each nipple and pull his cock into your mouth.

4 Use suction. Start at the head and go all the way down to the base of his cock and all the way back up and over the top.

5 Occasionally, pull him forward into your mouth with two hands cupped over his ass.

6 Just suck and twirl your tongue around the head of the penis. Make sure you get the underside of the head, one of the most sensitive spots.

7 Direct him to put his legs around your neck so you have his package directly in front of you. Put his penis in your mouth and simply press your tongue to the roof of your mouth and occasionally swallow.

8 Run your fingers through the crack of his butt cheeks. When you get to the base of his penis, try to go as deep as you can. When you have taken him in as far as you can, press the back of your tongue to the roof of your mouth. This is the French Press.

♀ WHY IT WORKS FOR HER

★ You see the erotic silver lining in everything. Wherever you go, sexiness goes, even to your workouts. You no longer have to worry about being sexy or not—with each erotic action, each erotic thought, you are it.

♂ WHY IT WORKS FOR HIM

★ Incentive! Incentive! You give him inspiration and an unforgettable workout session. Trainers charge big money to work with a client. I think you will get him better results.

RELATED MOVES

★ With every exercise, you should work the opposing muscle. For this exercise, the opposite would be a push-up. Have him do push-ups from the missionary position. Proper push-ups include a straight core. His body should look like a rising and lowering plank. With each successful push-up, give him a little love spank on the ass.

★ Another variation would be that each of you identifies your own personal goals (e.g., ten pull-ups). Each time one of you achieves their personal goal, he or she is rewarded with sexual favors. No penalties. Only positive sexy associations allowed.

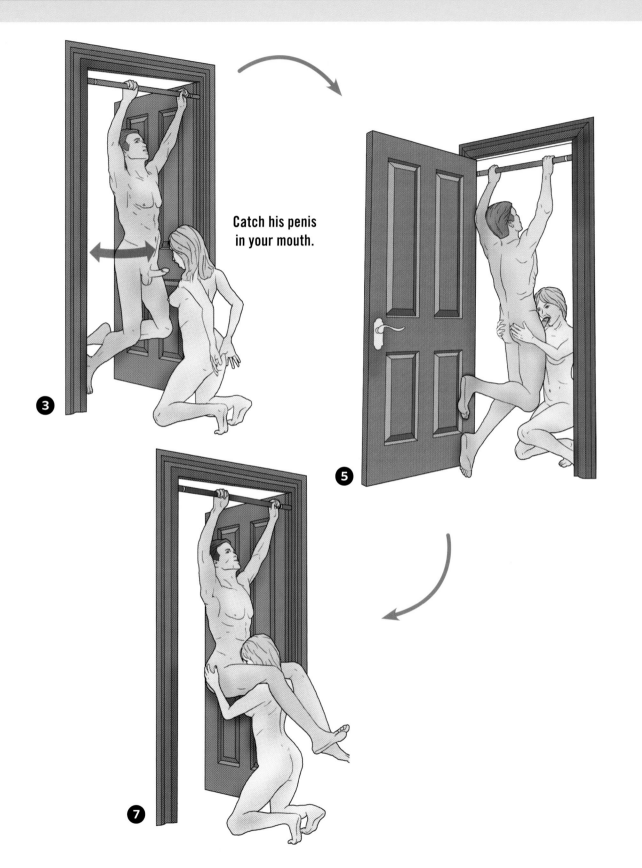

Catch his penis
in your mouth.

3

5

7

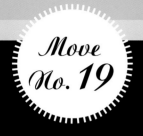

Move
No. 19

CLEAN YOUR PLATE

Have you made the deal that you would do the cooking if he did the cleaning, only to find you're still doing both? Annoying! Besides, it's boring.

This position will have him rolling up his sleeves and scrubbing the dishes without your having to say a word.

The Move: Clean Your Plate

THE PREPARATIONS

★ Unless you have the time and cooking feels like a sensual and sexy experience, for example, as seen in the movie *Like Water for Chocolate*, buy takeout and empty it into dishes. Why expend all your good sexual energy on making a food that you likely won't eat much of anyway?

THE LEAD-IN

After you finish your meal, lick your lips suggestively. Lick your fingers one by one. Lick his fingers one by one in a way that suggests that you want to lick his whole body, including his mouthwatering, lip-smacking penis.

While he loads the dishwasher, unzip his pants and begin licking in broad, plate-cleaning strokes up and down his cock.

Wrap the dishtowel around his neck and gently pull him in for a kiss.

Now, wrap the dishtowel around his waist and pull him in, rubbing your vulva against his cock. (You are, of course, not wearing panties.)

Lasso the towel around his waist and guide him to the stacks of dishes.

You are a woman who knows what she wants and how to get it. But he may begin to seduce you, maybe by kissing your neck. Hold up! Don't give in so soon. There is work to be done.

Reach for the dessert spoon. Give him a lick. As you pull the spoon away from his mouth, replace it with your lips.

Look at him, deep throat the spoon, moan, and smile. Ask him if he liked dessert.

Holding on to his waist, slide down his body to the ground. Assume the kneeling position.

Tell him that you need to lick his cock clean. Unzip his pants, reach in, and rub the tip of his cock, lathering him up with his own sweet pre-cum.

SEX FACTS

- The AOL Health/*Glamour* Men's Sex Survey asked men, "If your girlfriend could be good at only one of the following, at which would you want her to excel?" Forty-eight percent responded oral sex, 45 percent said cooking, and 7 percent said sports. (Oral sex wins!)

- Heavy foods like pastas, meats, and high-fat foods require more energy to digest, sending both of you into a food coma. Think sex and plan light meals that will keep your energy levels high.

THE SEXPERT SAYS

From the research, it looks like cooking is a close second to oral sex. The men were probably really hungry when they filled out this survey. How many times have you heard of a relationship in trouble because she wasn't a top chef? Invest your energies in the sex and go for his favorite takeout. Do you think he would complain about paying a few dollars one night a week so he could see you feeling happy, sexy, rejuvenated, and wanting sex with him?

★ The Main Act

1. When you have him in this position, ask him to help you with the dishes. No, not later, now.

2. When he laughs and gives in (and he will), give him a good association with soapy dishpan hands. Taste his balls with your tongue. Mmm. His testicles are a good starting point, and beginning here helps ensure that they don't get overlooked and go uncleaned.

3. Twirl your pointed tongue around his balls in circles, round and round. Switch to counterclockwise.

4. Gently glide your finger from his perineum up the seam of his balls.

5. With a flat, loose tongue, move your way up the shaft and occasionally over the head. Look up to see him when your tongue hits the head of his penis.

6. Place a cupped hand on his balls, gently pulling down.

7. When saliva pools up in your mouth, drool it onto his cock. Make eye contact with him and then slowly pull away, creating a string of saliva.

8. Return your lips to his balls, adding a slight suction. When he gets into that rhythm, introduce the twirling of your tongue to the suction.

9. Give him long, broad, wet strokes to the shaft and over the top of the head. The idea is to make this really wet, so if you need to add tasty lube, do.

10. Place a hand on his balls and your mouth on his cock. Cover your lips and suck as you move your head back and forth.

11. "Pop" his penis by placing it to the inside of your check and then gently but rather quickly pulling it out with your hand. It should make a slight popping sound, similar to the sound you made as a kid when you did it with a finger.

12. When you are ready for him to come, run your tongue over the top, as you suck and twirl your tongue to his orgasm.

♀ WHY IT WORKS FOR HER

★ You: a sexual diva and a playful sex kitten, with a clean kitchen.

♂ WHY IT WORKS FOR HIM

★ This is the most fun he has had washing dishes, and maybe even the most fun he has ever had, period. The more you do the "clean your plate" position, the more help you will get in the kitchen, and the more fun you will have doing your basic household chores.

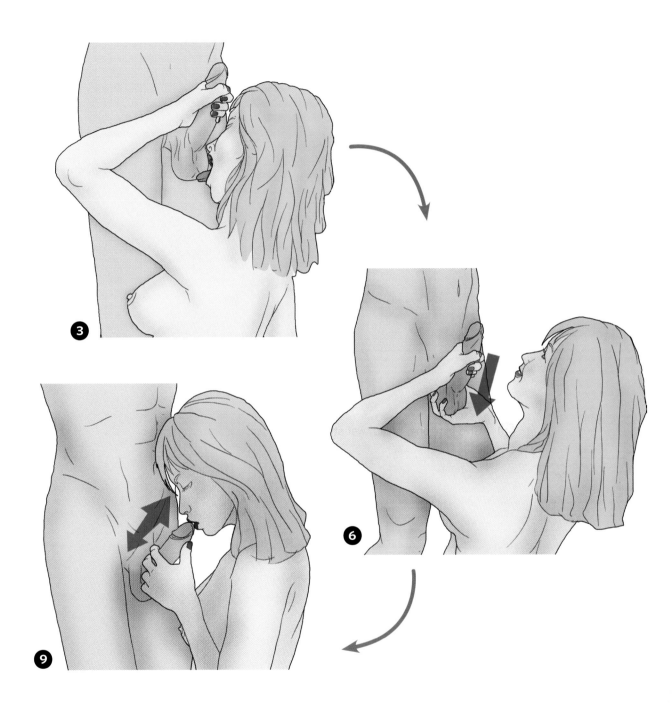

RELATED MOVES

★ Pull out all the utensils to whisk his nipples, baste his butthole, and bring the wooden spoon down on his ass. Yeah, baby! You're ready for your own show.

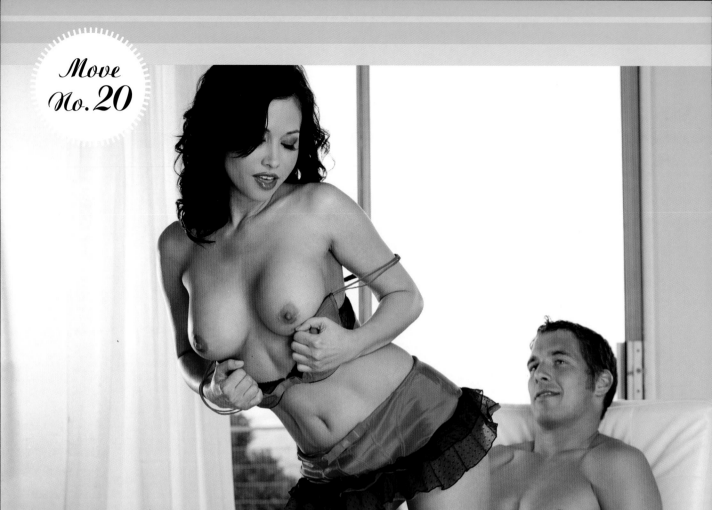

 # THE GLORY HOLE

Until now, glory holes were only known in gay bars and other gay hot spots. Give him the thrill of an anonymous heterosexual blow job by his favorite dancer.

The Move: The Glory Hole

THE PREPARATIONS

★ Your first mission is to figure out how high his penis is from the ground (this is probably one penis measurement he doesn't have).

★ The next time you are in a standing, fully naked embrace, identify where the base of his cock is in relation to your body. Does the base of his cock come to your waist, hipbone, belly button, clitoris—where?

★ Hang a white or light-colored sheet from a beam, room separator, hallway, or curtain cable.

★ Identify where his penis would be if he were standing up against the sheet and draw a circle. This circle will be the entrance for his penis and balls, so make it bigger than it needs to be.

★ You can keep the sheet hanging. Simply lift the sheet, fold it in half, and cut a half circle. Unfold it for your full circle.

★ Choose some music that helps you feel sexy.

★ In a full-length mirror, practice making some basic hip rolls and arm movements and shedding your clothing several times before the event.

★ Place a lamp on one side of the sheet, behind your dancing "stage," and a chair on the other side of the sheet. This is where he will sit.

★ Choose a G-string and clothing that you can take off in layers (e.g., wraps, button-down shirts).

★ Use a fragrance to arouse the senses.

THE LEAD-IN

Invite him to come to the bedroom for a special surprise. When he arrives, welcome him to the club, show him the glory hole, hand him a stack of singles or Monopoly money, and explain that there is no touching through the sheet.

If he likes the dance, he drops some bills to the ground. When he likes a particular dancer, he puts his penis in the glory hole and hopes she will notice him.

THE FOREPLAY

① Warm him up with a lap dance. Lead him to the chair behind the sheet and place his hands by his side. Remind him that he cannot touch you during the lap dance.

② Kiss him and move in close to rub your chest against his. Gaze into his eyes and smile as you think sexy thoughts. Put your leg on the arm of the chair and run your fingers along the inside of your thigh. When you get to your panties, pull them aside for a peek at your pussy. Place your finger over your clit and give it a little rub.

③ Change positions so you are kneeling over him as if he were going to spank you. Tilt your pelvis down so your clit is rubbing on his leg and tilt your pelvis up so your back is arched and he can really see the curve of your ass in the G-string.

④ Tell him that you need to go, but you hope that he will stay for the dance.

★ The Main Act

1 Go behind the sheet and dance around slowly to your music, removing layers of clothing. Allow your eyelids to fall in a relaxed gaze, feeling the music as it guides you to do moves that you may not otherwise do. Affirm to yourself that you are a free, beautiful, sexy goddess. Dance like you would if no one were watching. Dance as if you were in the shower and the sheet was a shower curtain.

2 When he puts his penis in the glory hole, dance by it once or twice, brushing up against it or blowing your warm breath on the head of it in a flirty tease.

3 Just when he thinks he is getting a BJ, pull away, and lay on the floor so he can see you spreading your own legs, massaging your breasts, and rubbing your clit. Carry on until you see some bills hit the floor.

4 When he pays up, place his delicate balls in one hand and lightly lick his cock as if it were a lollipop that you are savoring.

5 Get down to business by doing a sucking motion from the tip of his penis all the way down to the base and back up again. Do this move several times.

6 Move into a deep throat, pursing your lips and going all the way down to the back of your throat. Wrap your thumb and forefinger around his penis between your lips and the base of his cock. This modification will give the feeling of tightness on the shaft and allow for a greater sense of depth than no woman could possibly ever achieve.

7 If you can't deep throat, do an almost-deep throat (which is detailed more in my BJ book). Basically, put the back of your tongue to the roof of your mouth. When his penis enters, he will feel as if he were tapping the back of your throat.

8 Add speed, suction, and tongue twirls to the head on the out pull as you bring him to orgasm.

♀ WHY IT WORKS FOR HER

★ This night is going to end and the sun is going to rise in the morning, but your confidence will live on throughout the day.

♂ WHY IT WORKS FOR HIM

★ Men love attention, especially sexual attention. With the Glory Hole BJ, he gets sexual attention, a sense of mystery, and an amazing blow job all at the same time.

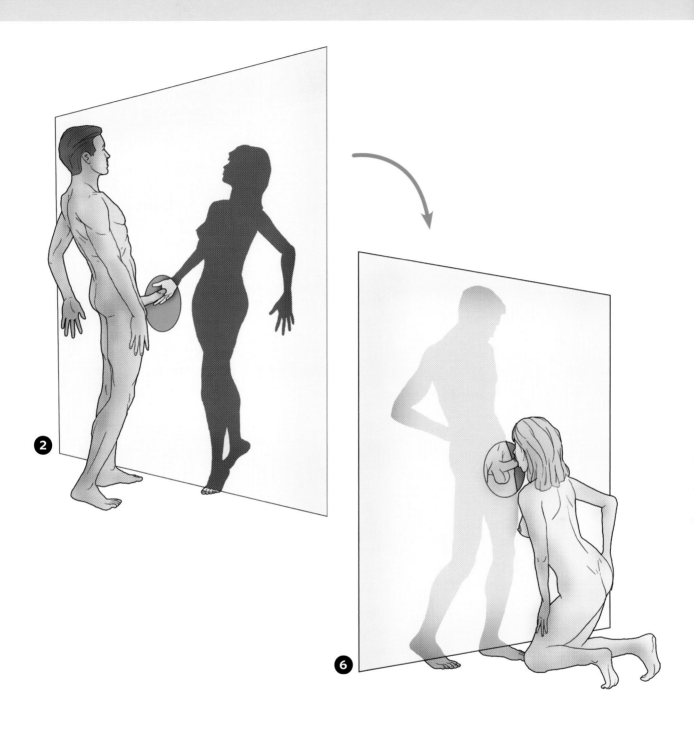

SEX FACT

According to the MSNBC/*Elle* survey, 32 percent of women who cheated said the reason for their actions was that they wanted reassurance of their desirability, and 47 percent of the men who cheated wanted more sexual variety.

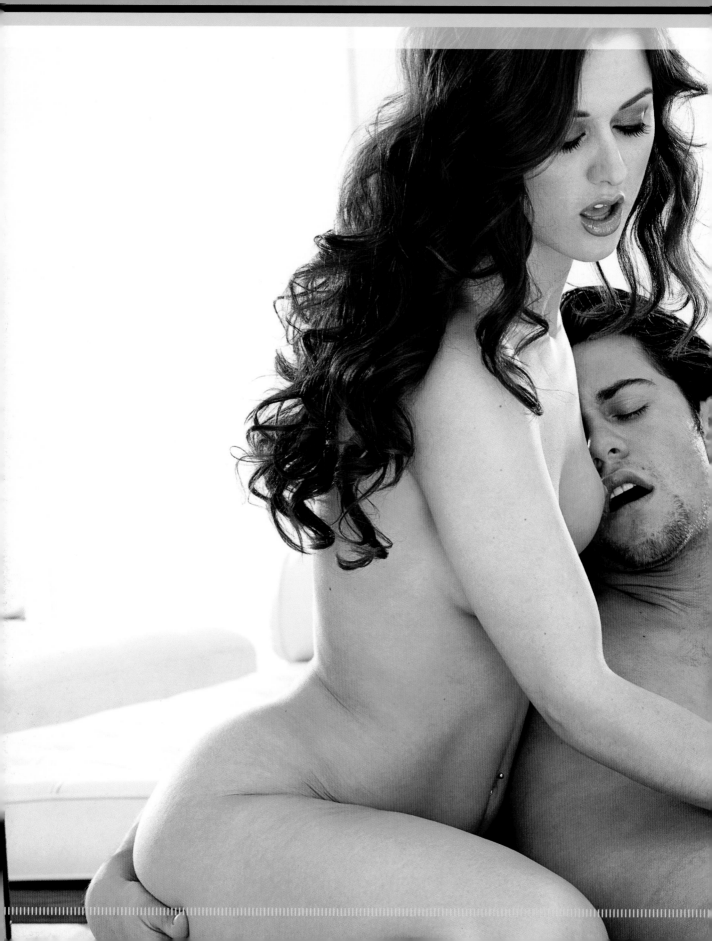

Hand Jobs

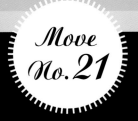

Move
No. 21

AMBISEXTROUS

Are you single-handedly making love to your partner? I mean, do you only use your dominant hand during sex? If so, learning to be Ambisextrous has its benefits. When you touch your lover with a nondominant hand, you can access different angles and positions. Every great masturbator and most men know that the feeling is different if you give yourself a lefty or a righty. I bet your lover knows it, too.

Have fun with this challenging position while you sharpen your skills at the same time.

The Move: Ambisextrous

THE PREPARATIONS

★ Practice pleasuring yourself with your nondominant hand. Notice the nuances and how different it feels. Some say it doesn't even feel like your hand at all, making your fantasies more believable.

★ Feeling awkward and uncomfortable is part of this position—just like that new pair of hot shoes felt awkward the first time you put them on, but after you pranced your sexy little self around in them, they felt normal and maybe even comfortable. My point is, don't give up during the awkward feelings. They are normal and part of the process.

THE LEAD-IN

Ask your guy if you can give him a lefty (or righty, if that is your nondominant hand) as you reach for his penis. Guide him to the bed. Lie him down on his back.

THE FOREPLAY

①   Do everything opposite. If you usually start with a kiss to his lips before making your way down his body, start today with a kiss to his feet, working your way up the nondominant side, of course.

|||||||||||||||||||||||||||||||||||||||||||||||||||||||||||||||||||||||||||||||||||||||||||||||||||||||||||||||||||||||

SEX FACT

According to the Askmen.com survey, 34 percent of men reported that they would like their partners to be more into sex in general.

|||||||||||||||||||||||||||||||||||||||||||||||||||||||||||||||||||||||||||||||||||||||||||||||||||||||||||||||||||||||

THE SEXPERT SAYS

Learning specialists say that if you want to stimulate the left (logical) side of your brain, you should use your right hand for tasks. Likewise, if you want to stimulate the right (creative) side of the brain, you should use your left hand for tasks. Now why shouldn't those "tasks" be sexual in nature? Gives a whole new meaning to learning, doesn't it?

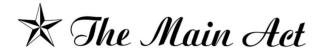

★ The Main Act

1 When it comes to hand jobs, wetter is better, so get some lube or go for the saliva.

2 Sit beside him so your nondominant hand is closest to his cock. Wrap your palm around his shaft and place your thumb over the head as if his penis were a joystick with a "shoot" button on the head. (For some men, it is.)

3 Stroke him straight up and down to start finding a rhythm. Play with the pace and pressure. Momentarily run your thumb over the head. Pet, pat, and pull his balls or run your fingers through his pubes with your dominant hand.

4 With each lefty stroke, notice the awkward feeling and keep going with the stroke until you either become fatigued or comfortable. Either one is great news. It means you got it and next time around will be super easy.

5 Now, you are going to switch positions and in the process you are going to give him a hot shot of your bodacious butt. Still by his side, scoot down and thrown one leg over this body, so you are facing his penis. He should be looking right at your ass. Put your weight on both knees and your nondominant hand on his balls, massaging your way up to his cock.

6 Stroke him, palms facing you, rubbing your thumb over the ridge of the underside of his penis. Keep your butt punched out and every once in a while turn back and check to see if he likes the view and all the little twists you are treating him to.

7 Spread your knees a bit, tilting your pelvis back and forth so you can rub your clit against his stomach or chest, boosting your own bliss.

8 Put your hands to the ground and lean your weight forward on your elbows, look between your legs and back your ass up closer and closer to his face. Know that he loves it! If you are feeling extra wild, tell him to kiss, lick, spank, or bite your ass.

9 From this elbows-to-the-ground position, most of the action is in your left wrist moving up and down, altering pressure and speed, and the fingers of your nondominant hand gliding over and caressing his balls. Combine the ambisextrous forces as you lead him to cosmic orgasm.

♀ WHY IT WORKS FOR HER

★ Personal growth fanatics will love Amibisextrous because you are constantly pushing your limits and making the uncomfortable comfortable, doubling his orgasmic pleasure.

♂ WHY IT WORKS FOR HIM

★ Two hands really are better than one, especially if they are both skilled. This fresh position hits new spots and keeps him not knowing what to expect.

★ And he is going to love the booty shots. The show from this position is off the charts.

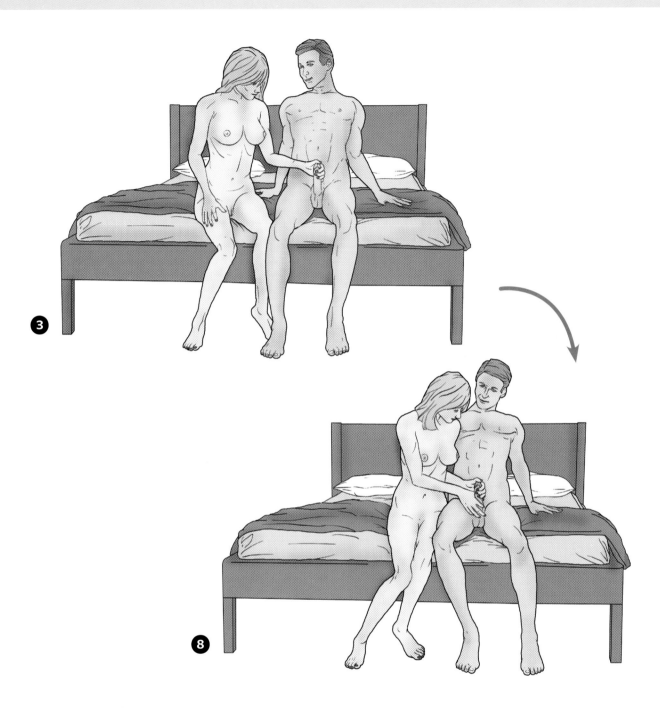

RELATED MOVES

★ Adopt a character. Again, your touch will feel different even to him, maybe even like a different woman. This could be your chance for a fun, safe, and hot erotic exploration together. Blindfold him and wear different perfume and attire that fits the character.

★ Give him a little mouth action, or at least some teasing warm breaths, especially when you are face-to-penis on your elbows.

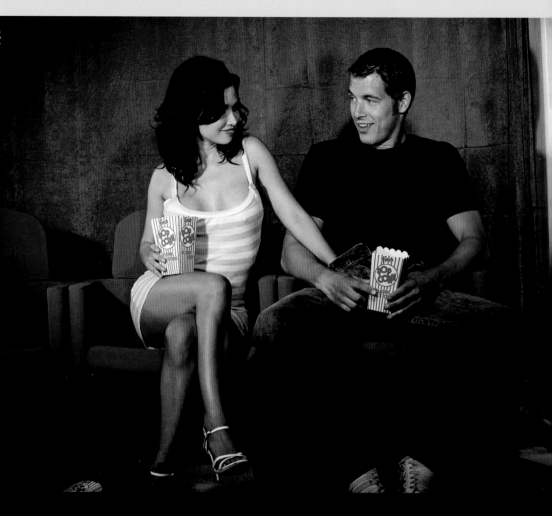

 # ★ ROMANCING <u>THE</u> BONE

This is as close to the action as you're going to get; it's your ticket to the best hand job

around. The movie hand job only works in a near-empty theater (or your home theater).

Choreograph the pace of your stroke to the film. What does a car chase scene feel like?

A romantic comedic scene? A horror scene?

The Move: Romancing the Bone

THE PREPARATIONS

★ Search the movie listings for a movie time and location that is not very popular. If possible, choose a movie with a lot going on. Action movies are known to have death, drama, and sex, which coincidentally release testosterone, which contributes to an erection.

★ Pack a plastic bag.

★ Order the largest bucket of popcorn. Cut or puncture a hole in the bottom with your finger. Empty the popcorn into the plastic bag for now.

★ You are going to have to sneak in some lube for this hand job. (Movie vendors have not caught on to this big money-making opportunity yet.) However, if you are in a pinch, there is always saliva.

★ Learn a little bit about screenplay storylines. Watch a movie and identify the beginning, middle, and end of the story; identify the conflict, the protagonist (good guy or hero of the story), and antagonist (bad guy); identify the climax (peak) and resolution of the story (how the story ends). After you've identified a basic storyline, match the emotions of the movie with a touch.

THE LEAD-IN

Tell him about the movie you would like to see and ask him if he'll take you.

THE FOREPLAY

① When you sit down, do the classic yawn and stretch your arm over his shoulder. Give him a big smile. He will smile back, without any knowledge that this will be the most memorable movie he has ever seen.

② Snuggle with him and feed him popcorn.

③ When the theater goes dark and the previews begin, turn up the flirting with kisses, blows, sucks, bites, and nibbles to the lips, neck, and ears.

④ Glide your fingers around the band of his pants, suggesting that you want in. Touch his crotch and give him a rubbing preview of what is to come through his pants.

⑤ Put a sweatshirt in his lap to cover the indecency that is about to take place. Unzip his pants and pull out his penis.

⑥ Put the popcorn bucket on his lap and pull his penis and balls through the hole you've made.

★ The Main Act

1. Using a soft, steady hand, reach down into the bucket to find his cock. Avoid touching the head of the penis at first, especially if it's a long movie.

2. Start by giving stimulation to his balls. Run your index and pointer fingers around one, then the other.

3. That was just the introduction of the movie. As the storyline develops, lube your hand and get down to business.

4. Sit close to him so you can hear his breath or put your hand on his heart or pulse to identify where his arousal level is. As a man becomes more aroused, his heart rate and breathing naturally become more rapid. Lighten or deepen your stroke in time with the scene and his natural rhythm.

5. Begin stroking his shaft in long, slow strokes.

   A. Match the movie scene: if there is a stalking scene, move your fingers to the head and lightly tap with one finger or squeeze the penis as if it were a beating heart.

   B. When there is a suspenseful scene, stop all sensation. Resume when the action does.

   C. During a car chase, do short quick and long quick strokes.

   D. For romantic scenes, do a twist and occasionally run your hand over the top. They love that.

   E. When there is a sex scene, follow the lead of the lady in the scene. For example, if she is teasing, tease the cock.

6. When you reach the climax in the movie, bring him to a climax in his seat, using all the techniques at your disposal—timing, pressure, speed, and lubrication.

♀ WHY IT WORKS FOR HER

★ We love to go to great lengths to prepare a delicious meal for him, a true experience. But you have already done that. This is not only a gift to him, but also to yourself. Stretch and expand your boundaries—and gain a better understanding of a movie plot.

♂ WHY IT WORKS FOR HIM

★ "More than a movie" is the simple slogan here. It's hot to know that your partner takes extra measures for you to experience something special.

RELATED MOVES

★ People usually do what they like done to them, regardless of the fact that he has a penis and you a vulva. Have him go in your pants and mirror what he does.

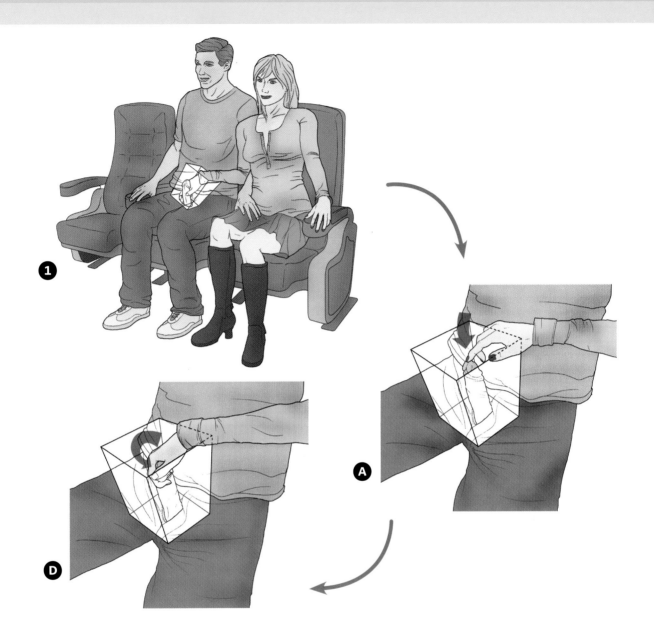

THE SEXPERT SAYS

To help him get more of a movie experience, use one of these techniques to help him last a bit longer:

★ **Cease sensation.** When you know that he is approaching orgasm, but obviously before the point of no return, simply ceasing sensation to the penis and putting focus somewhere else will help prolong the experience and keep him in the state of arousal.

★ **Gently tug on his balls.** Testicles will naturally rise prior to ejaculation. Gently tugging will help prolong ejaculation.

★ **Put pressure on the perineum.** Although he will still orgasm and may be ready to roll over and go to sleep, it is a good technique if you want to avoid ejaculation and the extra cleanup in the movie theater.

HAND JIVE

Are you too tired for sex? Is the common cold, allergies, or a stuffy nose getting in the way of performing oral sex? Too messy to have intercourse while on your period?

Hand jobs are great for several reasons: they don't expend a great amount of energy, you can do them with a stuffy nose and still breathe, and there is relatively little mess.

In this position, he lies on his back, sunny side up. You sit facing him with your butt between his legs, right leg draped over his left, left leg draped over his right.

The Move: Hand Jive

THE PREPARATIONS

★ Stretch your hamstrings and lower back. Sit on the floor with your legs out in front of you slightly opened; bend at the waist, reaching forward to touch your toes.

★ Stretch your wrists. Turn your wrists clockwise, then counterclockwise.

★ Stretch your mind. Get into a generous place in your heart and mind. Meditate on thoughts like "It's better to give than receive" and "You get what you give." You don't have to believe or adopt this mind-set, but see the beauty and feel the positive emotions of generosity, gratitude, and abundance that come with giving without expectation of return.

★ Light a candle or turn on a night-light so you can see him.

THE LEAD-IN

The next time you hop into bed, kiss each other, and are about to roll over to opposite corners and go to sleep, turn around, snuggle up to him, and whisper in his ear what you want to do to his cock. Describe his cock in vivid detail.

THE FOREPLAY

①   Scratch his back, starting at the top. Give him long, slow, teasing scratches all the way down and back up again.

②   Reach down to his balls and glide your fingernails over them, giving a nice slow, gentle scratch.

③   Extend your tongue and flick it over his nipple. Flicking is a great time to connect eyes because you can turn your head and look up at him at the same time. Lick your way down to his penis.

THE SEXPERT SAYS

The first phase of the sexual response cycle occurs in the brain, the most important sexual organ. Describe the brain chemistry of the sexual response cycle. Why should you know this? You have heard of the 80/20 rule, right? When it comes to quickie sex, 80 percent of your time should be spent in the arousal phase and 20 percent in the act. This includes the time you invest in arousing yourself. If he sees you aroused, he will be turned on, too.

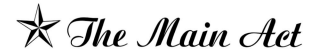

★ The Main Act

1 Give short sucks to the head of his penis, calling all the energy up his cock.

2 Allow your saliva to drip down his shaft and trickle onto his balls. Use the saliva to lubricate his penis, and give slippery glides to his shaft.

3 Using the thumb and forefinger of your left hand in the shape of an A-okay, glide your hand down to the base of his cock and hold it firmly. This will act as a cock ring and expose the nerve endings in the head of his penis. This technique works particularly well with the uncircumcised penis.

4 Continue stroking his cock up and down in a steady motion.

5 Occasionally, flick your tongue over the head of his cock, with the same playfulness you did to his nipples. While you are flicking, look up and make eye contact with him.

6 Twirl your finger around the head of the cock clockwise, then counterclockwise. This is a good time to watch him and be conscious of your energy exchange. As you generously give hand strokes, consciously visualize your heart opening up. Watch him and be aware of how his moans and facial expressions affect you. Where do you feel his energy landing on your body as he experiences you?

7 When you are ready for him to come, increase the speed of your stroke and add suction and swirls with your mouth to the head of his penis.

♀ WHY IT WORKS FOR HER

★ Sometimes you just don't feel like having intercourse or giving a blow job. You're not in that moment. But watching your partner come is satisfying.

♂ WHY IT WORKS FOR HIM

★ You are satisfying his carnal cravings and respecting your own limits—and everyone wins. Compromising is sexier than saying "not tonight, dear."

RELATED MOVES

★ Mouth-to-penis contact is optional, since this is a hand job, but the flicks of the tongue do not block your air passage or require much effort. They are more for psychological stimulation.

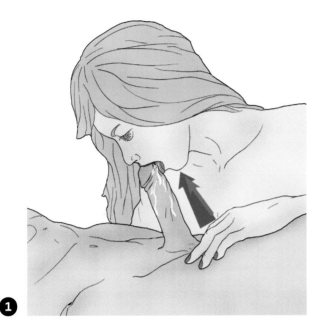

1

Glide hand up and down the shaft.

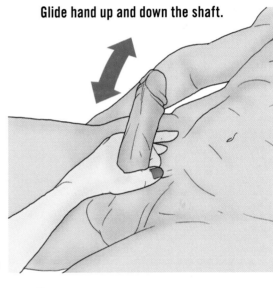

3

Twirl finger around head, swiching directions.

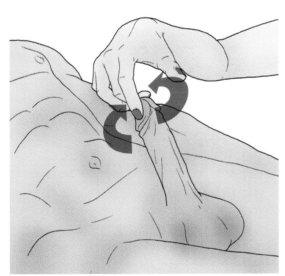

6

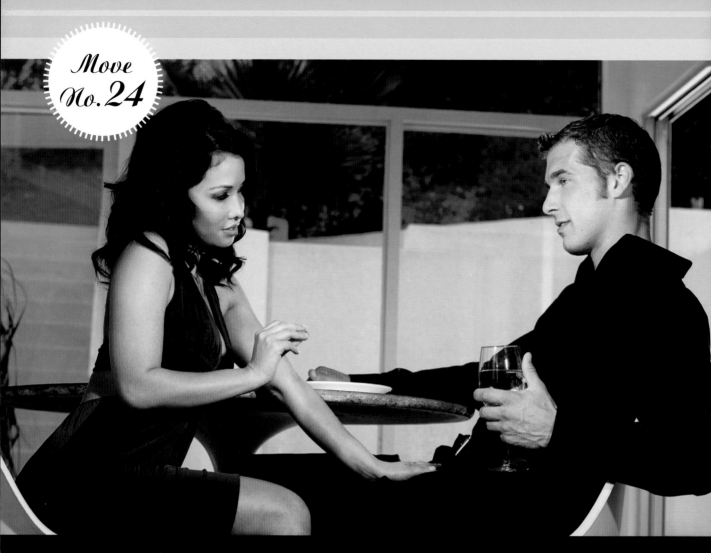

THE UNDER-THE-TABLE HAND JOB

You can do this one at an isolated small table in a very dark restaurant—or at home.

Drop your napkin. Unzip his pants on the way back up. While you're studying your menu,

pull out his cock. Play a little, put your hand back on the table, back under—and so forth.

The pauses will drive him crazy.

The Move: The Under-the-Table Hand Job

THE PREPARATIONS

★ Accept a lunch or dinner invitation from him, or ask him to take you out. If you can't arrange it for whatever the reason, set up your own little corner table at home.

★ Choose a place with tablecloths, preferably long tablecloths.

★ If having a glass of wine will help you relax and get out of your head, go for it. I am not suggesting that you drink yourself out of consciousness. Most of us are so self-conscious that we think everyone is looking at us. The truth is that most strangers are spinning with their own thoughts. They don't notice you at all.

Disclaimer: Public play can be exciting and highly erotic, but there can be legal ramifications, so be discreet.

THE LEAD-IN

Brush your foot up against his and giggle like a schoolgirl sharing a milkshake.

Feed him bites of your food and back it up with a sweet kiss, a taste of your dessert following each bite.

Take a few bites of your food. When it tastes especially good, moan with delight. After all, you are a sensual woman, and sensuality is about finding pleasure in life, including in this delicious meal.

THE FOREPLAY

① Start by dropping your napkin on the ground. As you pick it up, unzip his pants.

② Put your hand in his lap. Stroke his cock; making sure it is hard before going down is essential. Otherwise, you could be down there a long, long time.

SEX FACT

According to a MSNBC/*Elle* magazine poll, 38 percent of women said they think their partner wants sex more often, while 66 percent of men said they actually want more sex.

THE SEXPERT SAYS

Is there a perceived gap between what men and women want and what we think the other wants? Does your partner want more passion? That is usually one of the first things to fade in a relationship. You may say, "but we're best friends," or "we have a deep connection and passion/sex is not that important." Does he know this? And does he feel the same way?

★ *The Main Act*

1 Reach down and give that cock a hello with your hand. A smooth, soft touch says, "It's a pleasure to see you."

2 Starting at the base, turn your hand so your thumb is facing up and gently stroke down and up, working toward a gradual build. To do this, you will want to avoid the head of the penis.

3 Clumsy, sexy girl, choose another item to drop, perhaps a fork or an earring.

4 Take a deep breath and kiss him. Maintain eye contact as you're going down until your eyes pass the edge of the table, he is out of view, and you are looking at his cock.

5 Breathe a warm breath on his bare cock while you run your fingernails up his trousered legs. Pull out his balls and blow a warm breath on them, too.

6 When you come up, reach for his hand. Kiss, and suck his fingers as if his phalanges were his cock. I know it sounds silly and pornlike, but men love it.

7 Touch his balls. They might still be wet from the moisture of your breath. Gently circle them with your fingers and cup them with your hand, moving from left to right ball and then both at once. Gently lift and tug them.

8 Go up and down, giving him goodies. When you've dropped all of your silverware and half of your attire on the ground, finish him off.

9 Firm up your grip when at the shaft. On your way up, twist your hand and bring it over the head. When you go over the head, loosen up your grip so it is just a brush. He will moan. The head of the penis has many nerve endings, much like our clitoris.

10 Watch, feel, and listen. Watch his face, feel the pulse of his cock, and listen for his breath and his moans. Find a rhythm and finish him off with the Under-the-Table Hand Job.

♀ WHY IT WORKS FOR HER

★ You just created an immortal sex tale starring you. Whether you remain together or apart, this little erotic encounter will be celebrated for a long, long time.

♂ WHY IT WORKS FOR HIM

★ Food and sex in public—does it get better than that?

RELATED MOVES

★ Go to the bathroom and remove your panties. When you return, hug him from behind, draping your arms around him and dropping the lacy thong in his pocket.

★ Or, after you've removed your panties, put his hand in your lap. If this fun little adventure is turning you on, he will find his finger slipping inside from your wetness. Your wetness is a compliment to him and a celebration of your sexuality.

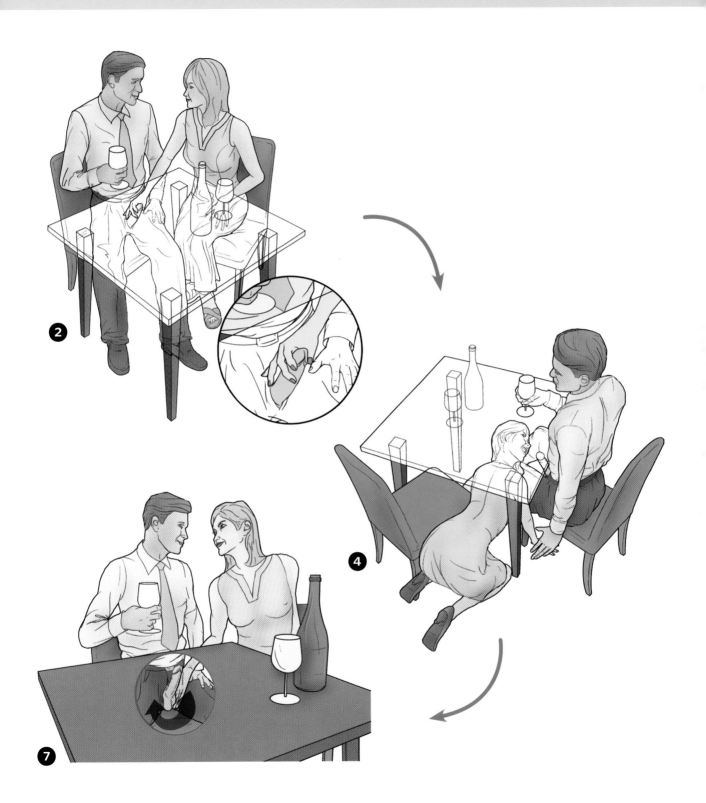

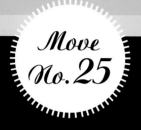

POWER LUNCH

"Oops, I dropped my napkin," you declare. When he goes to pick it up for you, he finds you spreading your legs open for him to see—and you're not wearing panties. As lunch progresses, occasionally reach under the table to stimulate yourself. He won't be able to take his eyes off your face.

The Move: Power Lunch

THE PREPARATIONS

★ Wear your best transparent sundress. No panties—or you can remove them before you show your world.

★ Shave or closely trim your pubic hair. You want to give him the best view.

Disclaimer: Public play can be exciting and highly erotic, but there can be legal ramifications, so be discreet.

THE LEAD-IN

Accept a lunch invitation or ask him to take you out to lunch. This could be with a new lover or a date with a longtime partner. It doesn't matter where you go, but wherever you choose, from here on out, this restaurant will be his favorite.

THE FOREPLAY

① Flirt with him.

② Look into his eyes and smile. Run your fingers through your hair, expose your neck, touch your leg, and brush your foot up the inseam of his pants.

③ Ask questions about him, lean forward, nod, and really listen to him. When he sounds like he is finished with his sentence, wait an extra ten long seconds, the Mississippi kind. Men often complain that they can't get a word in edgewise with a woman. This little gesture of listening helps him feel heard, appreciated, and comfortable with you.

④ Now ask him questions about sex. If this is a date with your new lover, you can start off small and ask him about his favorite position, or places he's had sex. If he is your established lover, ask him to describe what he would like you to try.

SEX FACT

Contracting (or tensing) certain muscles increases blood flow, and increased blood flow is part of arousal. Also, as orgasm approaches, men and women naturally tense up. Exaggerating the tension may help trigger and intensify orgasm.

THE SEXPERT SAYS

Men get pleasure from seeing their women pleased. In fact, many partners will climax when they feel their partners are close to orgasm. Making pleasure sounds sends signals to him. When you are approaching orgasm, tell him that you are coming, so he knows what brings you over the top.

Some women are too inhibited to be vocal during sex. If you are one of them, practice being vocal during masturbation. Imagine that your pussy is the instrument playing the melodies that are coming out of your mouth. I call this an "authentic allowing." Making noises during sex isn't exhibitionistic, although you may feel like it is when you're new to speaking/singing out. Doing this for the first time likely won't feel natural, but that is true for trying anything new for the first time. Practice brings a comfort level.

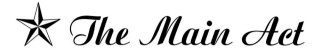 The Main Act

1 Capture his attention. When you have him, *hold* eye contact with him while you push the napkin off the table.

2 If he doesn't see that you deliberately pushed the napkin, declare, "Oops, I dropped my napkin." If he doesn't pick it up, ask him if he will.

3 When he leans down to pick up the napkin, spread your legs open just a bit so he can see your gorgeous pussy. He has no doubt that this is for him.

4 When he pops up with the biggest smile you have ever seen, resist the urge to talk. Don't say anything for a while. Just enjoy the energy radiating off him. Look how happy you made him with that little, itty-bitty gesture. Men are so easy to please and so very grateful for your erotic gifts. Let this be your first of many.

Disclaimer: Do not let him operate a motor vehicle or heavy machinery after this move!

5 Ask him how many fingers you are holding up. Ask him if he liked what he saw. Ask how he feels right now. Is he aroused? Is his cock hard? He may not be very articulate right now. That was the equivalent of looking at the sun, and he may need some time to readjust.

6 Lean forward across the table and kiss him. Whisper how much it turned you on to do that and see him being so turned on.

7 Take a deep breath and soften your face.

8 Reach into your pussy and offer him your finger to lick.

♀ WHY IT WORKS FOR HER

★ This is the ultimate "girl power" move. You will realize just what a beautiful, powerful piece of art you are. The anticipation of sharing your gift, the look on his face when he appreciates it, and the memories of the shared experience will be engrained in your mind for the rest of your life.

♂ WHY IT WORKS FOR HIM

★ Positions like the Power Lunch are what men wish, hope, and pray their girlfriends would do for them, but never do.

RELATED MOVES

★ With breathy whispers, tell him what you are doing. Are you circling your clit with your finger? Inserting it into your vagina?

★ Have him sit down beside you and let him touch the art.

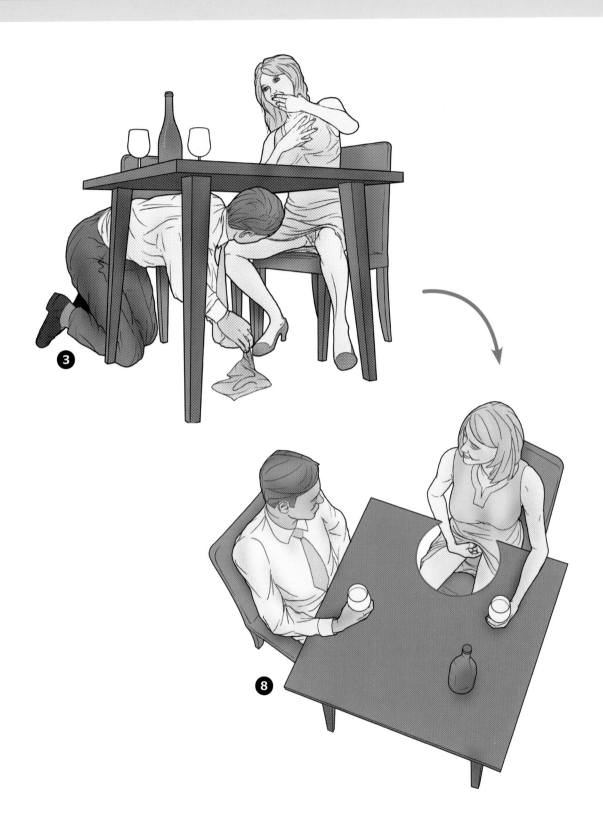

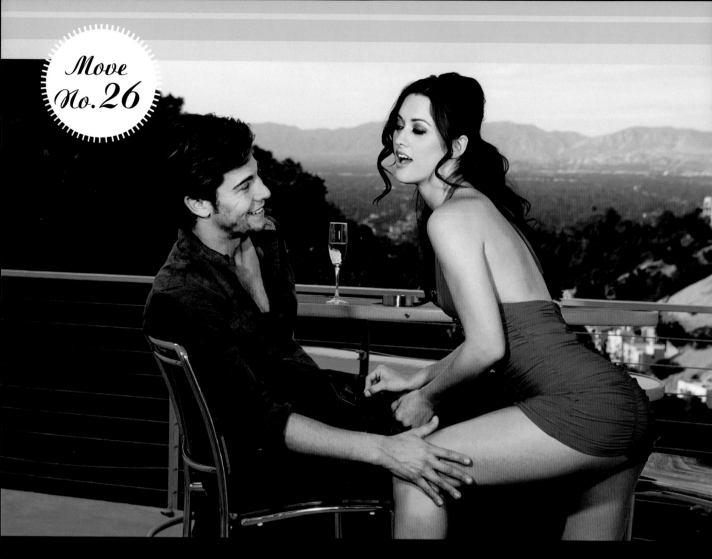

DANCING ON THE BARSTOOL

How many times have you been out dancing and thought, "Dancing is really similar to sex with clothes on." It's true: sexual energy is often built up on the dance floor by giving each other a clothed sex sample. Now that you have all that wonderful sexual energy built up, let's use it.

He sits facing the bar; you sit sideways facing him. He begins "dancing" in his chair in time to the music. You put your hand over his cock (kept inside his pants) and squeeze in time to his dancing. Finish in the restroom or the car.

The Move: Dancing on the Barstool

THE PREPARATIONS

★ Scout out a bar with a jukebox and ask him to take you.

★ Play a series of songs he likes and can dance to. Ultimately, when your hand is on his package, he will find his groove in this position, no matter what the song.

THE LEAD-IN

From the standing position, start rubbing your body against his in time to the music. Theoretically, this is dancing, but don't ruin it by asking him to dance, just act. Some men get embarrassed with the thought of dancing even if it is with the sexiest woman in the bar. If he says something like "I don't dance," reply with something like "We're not dancing; I'm just rubbing my body against yours, imagining that I am [pick one: a) being penetrated by you, b) fucking you silly while everyone watches, c) rubbing my clit against your cock]." Any one of these fantasy statements will capture and maintain his attention, so choose your own version, but notice that they all have sex in common.

THE FOREPLAY

① Even if he is game for the dance, describe the bump and grind as detailed above. Psychological stimulation is part of sex.

② Stroke his bulge with your clothed vulva and then your hand.

③ Celebrate his erection by talking about the hardness of his cock. Ask him if he is hard for you.

Disclaimer: Do not let him operate a motor vehicle or heavy machinery after this move!

||||||||||||||||||||||||||||||||||||||||||||||||||||||||||||||||||||||||||||||||||||||||||||||

SEX FACT

Men consider penis size the third most important feature for a man, while women rated it only ninth.

||||||||||||||||||||||||||||||||||||||||||||||||||||||||||||||||||||||||||||||||||||||||||||||

THE SEXPERT SAYS

Men love to talk about their erections with you. They are so proud of their cocks and they want you to be, too. They will say things like, "I get so hard for you." Or "Look what you do to me." The comments are often followed by a guiding of your hand to his penis. Celebrate his penis with him. Talking about his cock could be a way of initiating sex.

★ The Main Act

1. You have him in the mood. Sit him down so you are standing facing him with your dominant hand on his pants.

2. Your nondominant hand is holding a full drink. You don't want to be interrupted and possibly discovered by a bartender wanting to serve you another. (Or maybe you do?)

3. Never look at what your hand is doing; doing so will blow your cover. This is key.

4. Reach your hand into his pants and gently touch all around, down to his balls. Never ignore the balls. Become familiar with the area that you will be working. It is snug in there, but you can do it! I will tell you how.

5. Stand shoulder to shoulder, blocking eyes to your left. Pull his shirt from his pants so it covers any indecencies. If there is room on the waist band, put your hand down his pants and on his shaft (palm facing toward him).

6. Begin with a simple stroke up and down. Don't worry about being perfect at this point. He is probably still mid–prayer of gratitude for how lucky he is to be getting a hand job in a bar.

7. Snuggle up close to him and rub your shoulder to his, nibble his ear, and breathe warm breaths on his neck. Ask him if he likes what you are doing.

8. Occasionally slide your pinky finger over the top of the head of his penis, the most sensitive spot on most men. Once in a while, let the penis fall between your ring and pinky fingers, gently squeezing them together. On the downstroke, rub his balls with your thumb. Girl, you are good!

9. Take him into the restroom or out to the car to finish the job. (Tip the bartender to hold your drinks.)

10. As you stroke him, talk to him. Ask him how it feels.

11. Throw in some extras by running your thumb over the head of his penis, gently pulsing the shaft, or rubbing his balls.

12. Look at him and smile, lick your lips, and moan and breathe with him.

13. Finish him off with your best strokes or pull him into your mouth and give him an ending he won't soon forget.

♀ WHY IT WORKS FOR HER

★ The psychological stimulation of giving a hand job in public combined with beautiful people and the risk of getting caught will make for a quickie when you get home.

♂ WHY IT WORKS FOR HIM

★ There was just a party in his pants and he was the guest of honor. Of course he loves this position!

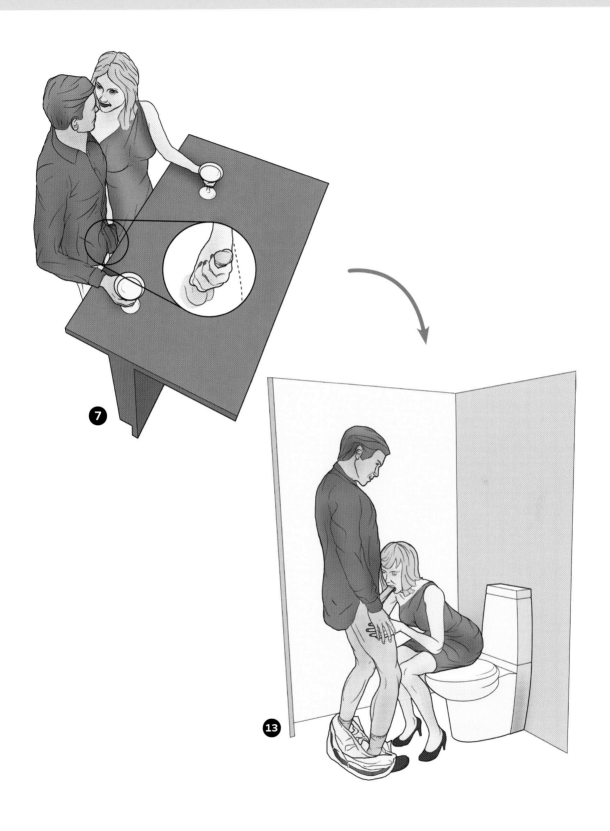

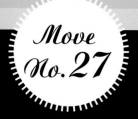

THE CELL PHONE HAND JOB

Surprise him with a sex toy—the Fleshlight or Sex in a Can. The Fleshlight is the number-one-selling male sex toy in the world. You will not believe the fleshy texture. Send him into another room with his new toy. Call him on your cell and tell him exactly how to stroke himself.

The Move: The Cell Phone Hand Job

THE PREPARATIONS

★ Looking like a large flashlight on the outside, the Fleshlight feels like a real vagina. It's perfect for traveling; it is his faux you. Purchase your Fleshlight either at a local sex toy store or online.

★ A little planning for this move is in order. Choose a weekend when he has few to no business calls.

THE LEAD-IN

Rubbing his cock with one hand and running your fingers through his hair with the other, whisper in his ear that you are hot for phone sex with him. And not some time in the future—*now*.

THE FOREPLAY

1. Hand him the Fleshlight and watch him open it.

2. Do a demo for him. First, put your own hand inside. Now it's his turn.

3. Reach into his pants. Touch his cock. Make sounds of approval. Praise his hard cock and his readiness to play.

4. Remove his pants. Lightly cup his balls with one hand. Gently stroke him from the bottom to the top.

5. Prop him up with pillows on the bed. Maintain eye contact while you slowly put the Fleshlight on his cock. Move it up and down. Watch him. At what point does he moan, shake, or shiver? Pay attention to what he likes.

6. Introducing the Fleshlight this way will create a positive association with you and his new toy. Psychologically speaking, the next time he uses the Fleshlight, he will remember this moment and it will not feel like he is jerking off into a can at all. . . . At least that is the idea.

7. Kiss his cock as you put on his underwear and place the phone under his balls. Say good-bye, and remind him that he should let the phone ring when he gets the call so he can feel the vibration. You love the idea of reaching out and vibrating his balls through the phone.

SEX FACT

If you are on the phone with a man and he asks, "What are you wearing right now?" There is a good chance one hand is holding the phone and the other is touching his penis.

THE SEXPERT SAYS

Sexually expanded is how you will feel after doing this move. Having phone sex is a great exercise or practice because it allows you to say and do things that you normally wouldn't if your lover were in the same room. Many women want to try phone sex, but they are not comfortable asking. There are probably hundreds of ways to ask, including "Do you want to have phone sex?" Here is one of many hot ways that you could propose the idea:

I am thinking about the last time I saw you and I am getting very excited. I thought about [describe the thought that turns you on—e.g., touching his balls and perfect cock]. Mmm. My [describe how the thought is physiologically turning you on—e.g., pussy is getting wet and my nipples are getting sensitive] just remembering you. Is your cock becoming hard listening to me right now? Do you want to touch it while I am on the phone with you now, and I'll touch myself?

⭐ The Main Act

1 Get comfy and naked in another room.

2 While you are calling him and vibrating his balls, get into the mood by doing what makes you feel sexy, touching yourself in all the right places. Be aware of your thoughts so you can share them with him during your phone-sex call.

3 When he picks up on the fourth ring, tell him how you were touching yourself and what you are fantasizing about. Get him to talk by asking him questions like: What are you thinking? Is your cock hard? Describe it to me. How are you touching it?

4 Begin to describe your vulva: the color of it, the feel of it, the smell, the taste. Draw out the delicious mental teasing. Describe the color, feel, smell, and taste of your clitoris, labia, butt, nipples, and vagina.

5 Say, "Pick up your Fleshlight. You are entering my vagina. Feel how tight and soft and warm my pussy is." Tell him the rules of the game. He can only change thrusting pattern with your permission. You dictate the pace, the pressure, the direction, and the technique.

6 If hearing him turns you on, encourage his grunts and groans with your own, raising the volume and the sexy vibes in the room.

7 Tell him to push his penis as far as he can into the Fleshlight. Describe the sensation on the head of his cock. Now, tell him to pull his penis all the way out so that he has to thrust between the fleshy lips to enter again.

8 Increase the pace of thrusting—and step up the fantasy action with it.

9 Have him put one hand on his balls or nipples, rubbing and stroking them as he continues thrusting with the other hand.

10 Allow him to do whatever he wants to orgasm as you describe your own.

RELATED MOVES

★ Pretend you dialed the wrong number. "I'm so sorry, I must have dialed the wrong number. You sound very nice and sexy. I'm all alone and feeling very sexy. Would you like to play?"

♀ WHY IT WORKS FOR HER

★ Women across the world breathed a sigh of relief when they discovered meals in a can. After all, you may not always feel like cooking a meal. The same is true with sex. You are both going to love pussy in a can.

♂ WHY IT WORKS FOR HIM

★ It's a great day: Phone sex and a sex toy for him. He will love his new phone lover and new toy, especially when you are not around.

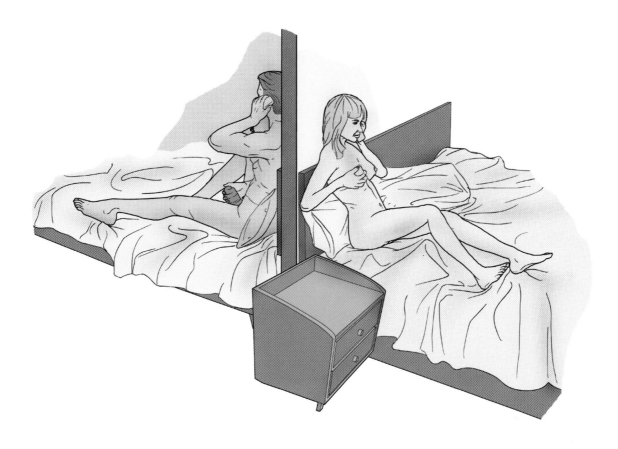

SEX FACT

According to Fleshlight.com, to clean the Fleshlight, "Simply rinse your removable Fleshlight sleeve with warm water from your sink and allow time for it to dry before storing. Do NOT use soap to clean your Real Feel Superskin sleeve. For tough cleaning, we suggest using a little isopropyl alcohol. To maintain that soft feel, sprinkle a liberal amount of cornstarch on the sleeve and shake off the excess powder. We do NOT recommend the use of talcum or baby powder. NOTE: Powdering an Ice Fleshlight masturbation sleeve with anything other than cornstarch will cause it to cloud over and lose its clear quality."

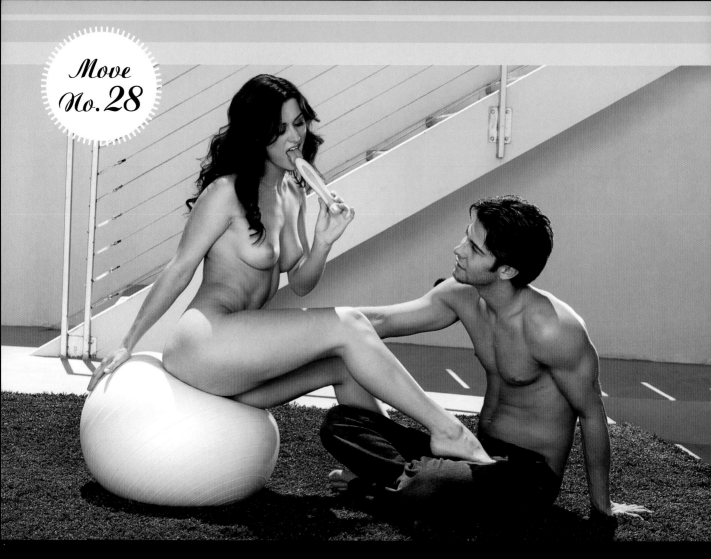

THE BOUNCING BALL HAND JOB

Ask him to straddle an exercise ball, belly down, leaning forward. He uses his hands to balance the ball while you reach between his body and the ball and give him a hand job.

The Move: The Bouncing Ball Hand Job

THE PREPARATIONS

★   Fill the ball with air. Make sure that the dildo and lube are within reach.

★   Unless you have experience on an exercise ball, you will want to practice.

THE LEAD-IN

Let him catch you doing your exercises naked on your exercise ball. Not the exercising type? You could roll it out to the TV room in the buff. Bounce on it a few times, really enjoying yourself as you watch whatever is on the TV. For some reason, no matter where in the world you are, men will see you bouncing on an exercise ball and imagine you bouncing on their penis. There is also an exercise ball with a dildo attached available at most online sex shops.

THE FOREPLAY

① Lean back on the ball, extending your arms over your head and to the floor and moving into a back bend. This position gives you a stretch and increases blood flow.

② Place the ball under your chest and roll it back and forth from chest to belly so your ass is up and facing him.

③ Rock the ball back and forth ever so slightly, occasionally stimulating your clitoris. Shorten the rocking motion so the focus is solely on the clitoris. Let him see you doing this.

④ Reach down and put your finger in your vagina and rub your moisture all around the inside of your labia majora (large outer lips).

⑤ When you are ready, insert the dildo and sit on the ball. Hold on to something like a table, couch, or his hands, so you can balance. When you are ready to go deeper with the dildo, thrust your pelvis forward so the dildo is pushed into you, or if you are feeling really randy, you can give it a little bounce as you are being penetrated.

SEX FACT

The angle at which you are stroking him will feel oddly familiar to him. That's because you are at the same angle he is when masturbating.

★ The Main Act

1 His turn. Get off the ball and walk toward him. He will likely be scooping his jaw off the floor after watching your show. Pull him to you by his hips and remove his pants as you kiss him passionately.

2 Have him lay facedown on the ball. Position it under his chest, with his knees on the floor and slightly apart.

3 Run your fingers between his legs and up to his balls. Circle his balls with your fingers, gently tugging. Slip your tongue up and just in between his butt cheeks. Squeeze, grab, and spank his ass, vibrating his genitals.

4 Get up close behind him and between his legs. As you get into position, brush your breasts against his ass and rest your head in the middle of his back. Reach your dominant hand down and start off at the base and with a loose hand. Work it upward toward the head of his cock. Squeeze lightly just under the head to release the pre-cum. Use the pre-cum as lubrication, slipping it over the head and down to the base of his cock. Continue with a few loose introductory strokes, sliding the penis between your thumb and forefinger. Fondle his balls with your other hand.

5 When you hear him moan or sigh, he's aroused. Keep up the stroke for a few more counts and then change it up by gradually picking up the pace. With the next moan or his sexy declaration that you are the bomb, change it up again by giving his cock a twist followed by gliding a hand over the head of his penis.

6 Need a break? Stop and let him thrust to find your hand. As he is searching, he's longing and developing a strong desire to penetrate. When you decide to stroke his cock again, let the head of his penis hit the palm of your hand. Form a loose-fitting fist. As he thrusts into the fist, perform a throbbing squeeze as if your hands were your vagina contracting in orgasm. Use your other hand to stimulate his balls. Bite, lick, and suck on his ass cheeks. Take him to orgasm.

♀ WHY IT WORKS FOR HER

★ You stretched, burned calories, and hopefully gave yourself a deep penetrating orgasm.

★ If you do the intercourse variation (see right), you will enjoy watching him maneuver as he hits all your deepest notes.

♂ WHY IT WORKS FOR HIM

★ He will never look at an exercise ball the same way again. He will forever have lusty images of you bouncing on your dildo and sense memories of the roaring orgasm you gave him while bent over in the "do me" position.

★ He will love, love, love resting on the ball while you stroke him to orgasm. It's very relaxing.

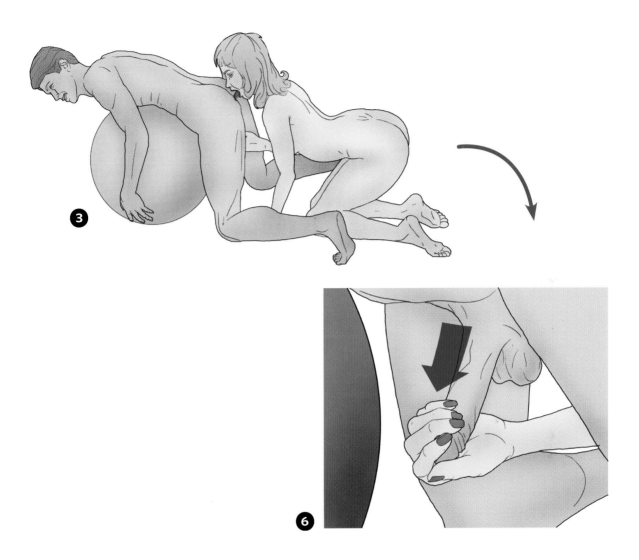

RELATED MOVES

★ Go down between the ball and his cock and give him some suggestive licks. Does he enjoy a P-spot massage? If so, this is the perfect opportunity.

★ This is a good position for anal play, but if neither of you are comfortable with that, open his legs and extend your tongue to reach his balls. Your nose will tickle his undercarriage and give him the psychological stimulation that you are going "balls out" on him.

★ Intercourse is amazing on the exercise ball. Lie on the ball so it rests between your lower and upper back, as if you were going to do sit-ups. He rests on his knees with your feet resting on his calves. He holds on to your breasts and pulls you in and out while twisting your nipples.

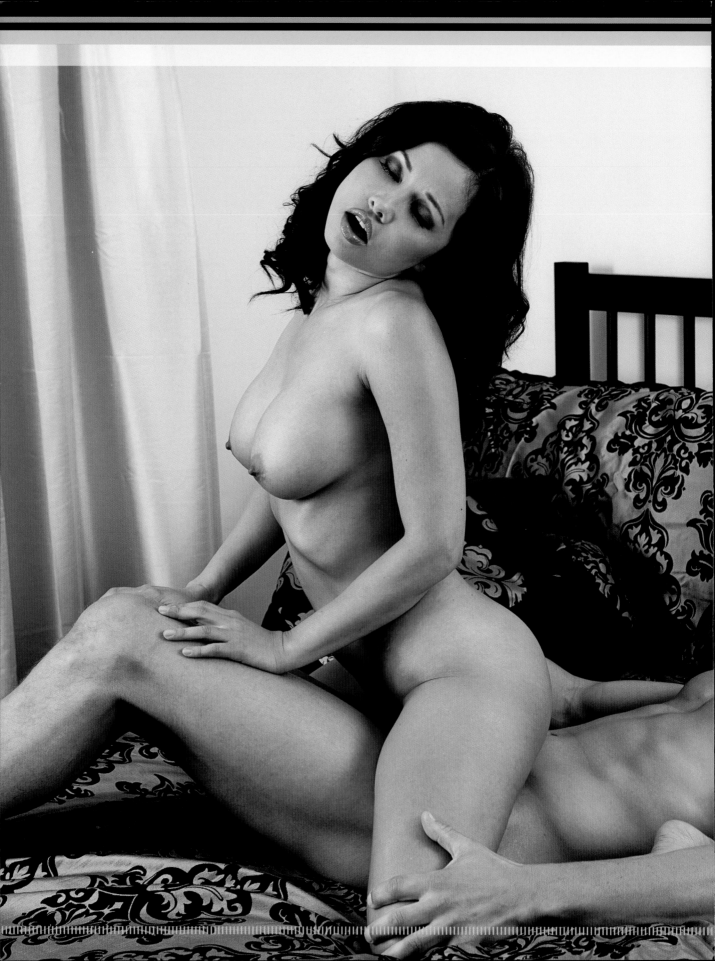

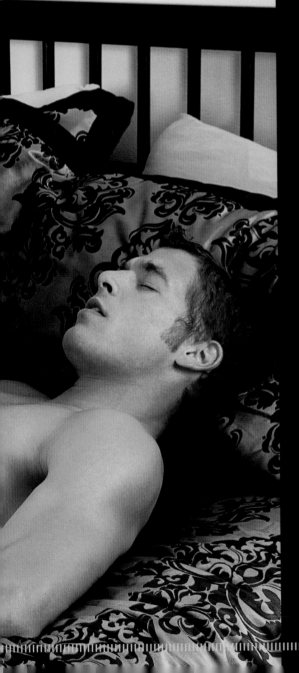

More
Happy Endings

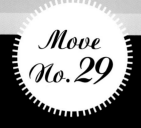

G-WORKS

Let him watch you shake and shiver in the blissful state of G-spot stimulation.

The G-spot responds to pressure and receives stimulation from the very large clitoral network, which consists of about 15,000 nerve endings that service the entire pelvic region. Access it by inserting a lubricated finger 2 to 3 inches (5 to 8 cm) along the upper side of the vaginal wall (tummy side) and pressing it toward the pelvis in a "come hither" motion. The G-spot will feel spongy when at rest and firm when aroused.

To stimulate the G-spot, pressure has to be applied *and* the woman has to be aroused.

The Move: G-Works

THE PREPARATIONS

★ Talk about the G-spot outside of sex play, like during dinner. Describe the last time he touched it, whether he was aware of it, and how it felt. Tell him that you would like to do more G-spot play. Guide him to your G-spot.

THE LEAD-IN

When you are ready to go full-on G-Works, take his hand and insert his finger, giving specific directions from there.

Explain the process: "Lube your finger and insert it about 2 to 3 inches (5 to 8 cm) inside of my vagina, and then move your finger in a 'come hither' motion toward the pubic bone. It should feel spongy when I am at rest and firm or rigid when aroused. The spot is the size of a quarter. You will want to press, grind, and rub on that spot. When I am close to coming, I will likely contract my muscles and feel like I need to pee, but it's not pee. This is where I might need some help to continue, as my natural reaction is to tense up and stop. It would be helpful if you encouraged me to relax continued stimulation, helped move my hips, or gave me leverage for thrusting so the stimulation continues through the peeing sensation."

Empty your bladder and lay down a towel in case you do ejaculate.

THE FOREPLAY

① The G-spot can be accessed from different positions. The keys are knowing your body well and keeping the location of the G-spot in mind. One little shift can make all the difference.

② When he inserts his finger, vocally guide him with cues like "That's it," "Faster," "Slower," or "More pressure." Always tell him if there is pain. When he get's it right, be sure to let him know.

③ You will know when he has hit the G-spot because it tingles, with surges running through your pelvis.

④ Contract your PC muscles for better stimulation *and* stronger orgasm.

⑤ Ask him to stimulate your clit and your anus and see where that takes you—probably over the top.

⑥ Remember to relax your body at orgasm and bear down or push through the "need-to-pee" feeling.

SEX FACTS

• Some women report that they can stimulate their G-spot externally by adding pressure directly above their pelvic bone.

• Some women ejaculate fluid through G-spot stimulation.

THE SEXPERT SAYS

Both men and women express body-image concerns, especially about their naked body. We can all benefit from exercise. When we look good, we feel good, and vice versa. Regular exercise will also help increase your endurance and muscle strength, which are both great for sex.

★ The Main Act

1 The woman-on-top position is a good place to start because you can take control and find your G-spot quickly. Start sitting up straight with a few quick gyrations, moving your pelvis back and forth. Lean forward and then backward to see what works for you.

2 Move into the reverse position and face his feet. Proceed slowly and carefully so you are stretched out on top of him—so you are both face to feet. Grab on to his ankles and slide yourself up and down. Move your hips around.

3 For more face-to-face intimacy, have him sit up and extend his legs in front and arms behind him. Bend your knees so they are close to your chest and your arms are behind you and between his legs. Rock yourself back and forth for a nice G-massage.

4 Move into the missionary position, and raise both legs up and back, until they are either on his shoulders or on his chest. Suggest that he kneel up against you to use your thighs as support. Grab on to his hips and guide him into you. Now, raise one of your legs and place it on his shoulder. Your other leg stretches out to the side, or you can bring it close to your body by bending at the knee. Place a pillow under your bum for better access and more comfort. Switch the legs back and forth and feel the head of the penis sweep across your G-spot.

5 Rest it up and move into a sideways spoon or onto your belly with your butt up, with shallow thrusts or circles (not in and out).

6 Switch to your back while he lies on top of you, sort of in a push-up position so as not to put all his weight on you but so he can still maneuver and thrust. Stimulate your clitoris and put direct pressure just above your pelvic bone with your fingertips or fist to externally massage your G-spot. Tilt your pelvis slightly so your rear is up.

7 Get on all fours so he can penetrate you doggy style. Keep your back arched slightly and lean forward into the bed without resting on it. Suggest that he pull on your hips as he thrusts in a downward motion all the way to orgasm.

WHY IT WORKS FOR HER

♀ ★ G-spot stimulation is particularly useful information if you would still like to have more orgasms but the clitoris is too sensitive.

WHY IT WORKS FOR HIM

♂ ★ He loves to see you receiving pleasure and he loves to hear and see you in orgasm, no matter where your stimulation is. The G-spot is different, and seeing you orgasm in many different ways is exciting.

RELATED MOVES

★ Imagine his penis shape and size, experimenting with different moves that best tap the spot. Remember to guide and give him feedback.

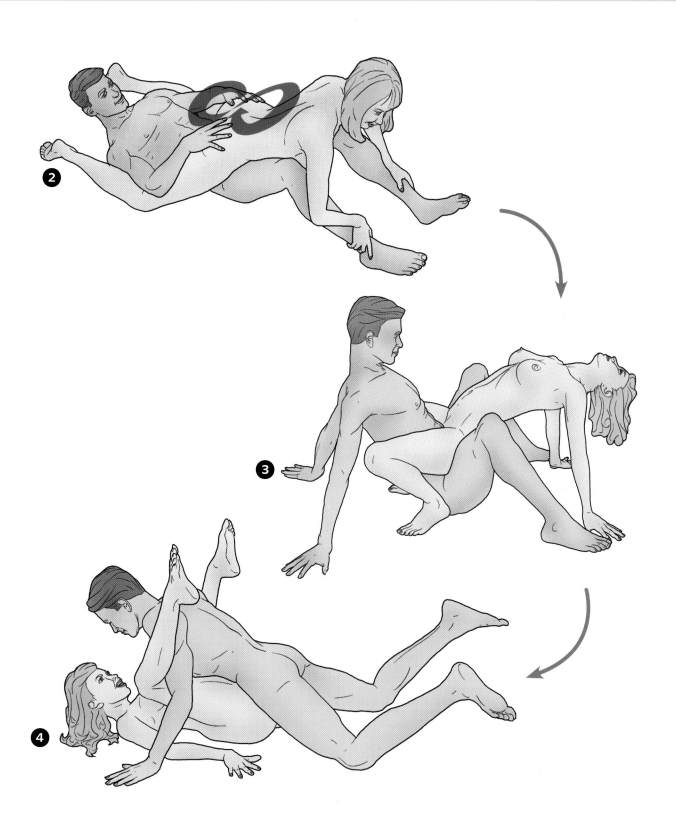

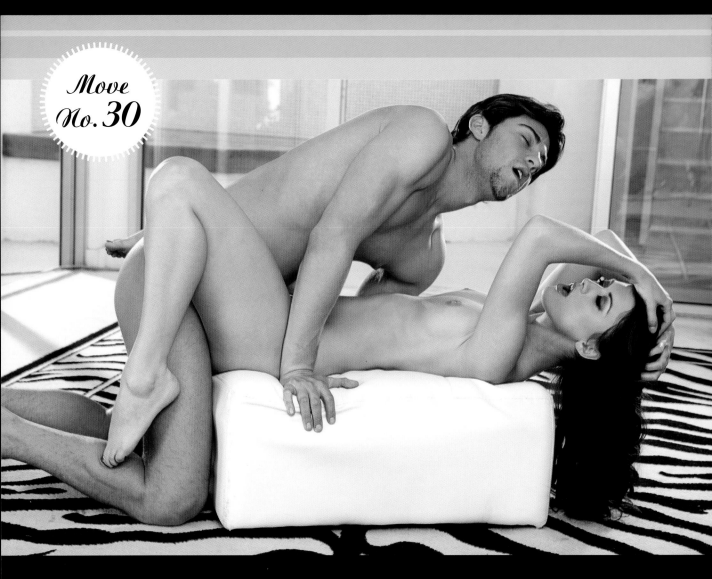

THE GRAND FINALE

This is the grand finale, or Tour de Sex, that you have both been dreaming about.

The Move: The Grand Finale

THE PREPARATIONS

★ Book your hotel room. Pack some lube in your overnight bag. Create a romping CD that makes you feel like doing it until the sun comes up.

★ After you check in at the hotel, go to the lobby restaurant. Sit across from him, drop your napkin, and do the Power Lunch (page 132). Let him see you pleasure yourself with your hand.

★ Pull up a seat next to him and give him the Under-the-Table Hand Job (page 128), but not to ejaculation.

★ Go back to the room. Hand him the bucket and ask him in your sweetest voice to get some ice cubes.

★ Put on a shirt that you can tear off your body, and put your Flower Power (page 144) strap-on dildo under your dress (optional).

★ Turn on the heater so you can prance around naked when the time comes.

THE LEAD-IN

When he comes back to the room, pull him inside and kiss him with his back against the wall. Men want to feel desired, so give it to him, girl.

THE FOREPLAY

① If you both enjoyed Flower Power, surprise him with your strap-on erection as you press your body against his.

② Rip off your shirt as you did his in Dressed to Thrill (page 70). While in the standing position, kiss, lick, and suck—and pull his clothes right off of him.

③ Get down on your knees. Put a few ice cubes in your mouth, spit them out, and put your mouth to his penis. Suck him with your cold mouth.

||||||||||||||||||||||||||||||||||||||||||||||||||||||||||||||||||||||||||||||||||||||||||||||||||||||||||||||||||

THE SEXPERT SAYS

Let all the sex and relaxation change your life. Women can really learn something from men in this area. Men don't feel guilty and don't need a reason to relax. When you reenter the world, think about how you will restructure your life so you do have time for sex and pleasure. It will only stick if you create the time and protect it.

⭐ The Main Act

1 Lift your leg up to his waist while you give him the Quiet Riot (page 78), pushing and thrusting with delight.

2 While he is still pressed against the wall, tie his hands behind his back as you did in Up Against the Wall (page 74), rub your Flower Power harness on him (since you forgot your toy pistol), and order him to give it to the naughty she-cop as you lead him to the dresser, where you do the Mirror Images (page 40).

3 Switch and move to the bed, where you give it to him in a subordinate position, all For the Love of Honey (page 94).

4 No coming yet! Stay at the height of arousal.

5 So you don't have a ball . . . but you do have an ottoman. Take him by the hand and rest him over the top. Lube your hand and stroke his cock from top to bottom as you use the other hand to massage his balls. Switch it up and lie over the ottoman, doing a back bend, opening yourself up in vulnerability so he can climb on top and access your G-spot with his penis.

6 Open the drapes a bit, or a bit more if you dare to be an exhibitionist.

7 Move to the bed and watch the sparks fly with G-Works (page 150).

8 Talk dirty and be as loud as you want because you can. If someone is unhappy, you will get a call. Otherwise, assume your neighbors are enjoying the sounds so much that they decide to have sex.

9 I dare you to make it twenty-four hours of sex, sleeping, sex, eating, and sex only. No phones, no television, no computers. Come back to join the world fresh and rejuvenated. Now that's a vacation!

♀ WHY IT WORKS FOR HER

★ You have just shown him—and, more important, yourself—how sexy you are when you can create the space. Keep your bags packed. I predict that you will have many more hotel overnights.

♂ WHY IT WORKS FOR HIM

★ He is going to love doing it in every square inch of the hotel room and having your undivided attention.

RELATED MOVES

★ It's all about the sex drugs. The neurotransmitter dopamine, released during orgasm, triggers a stress-reducing relaxation response that lasts up to two hours. Oxytocin, which kicks in about fifteen to twenty minutes after orgasm, plays a role in sleepiness, explaining the "roll over and go to sleep" response.

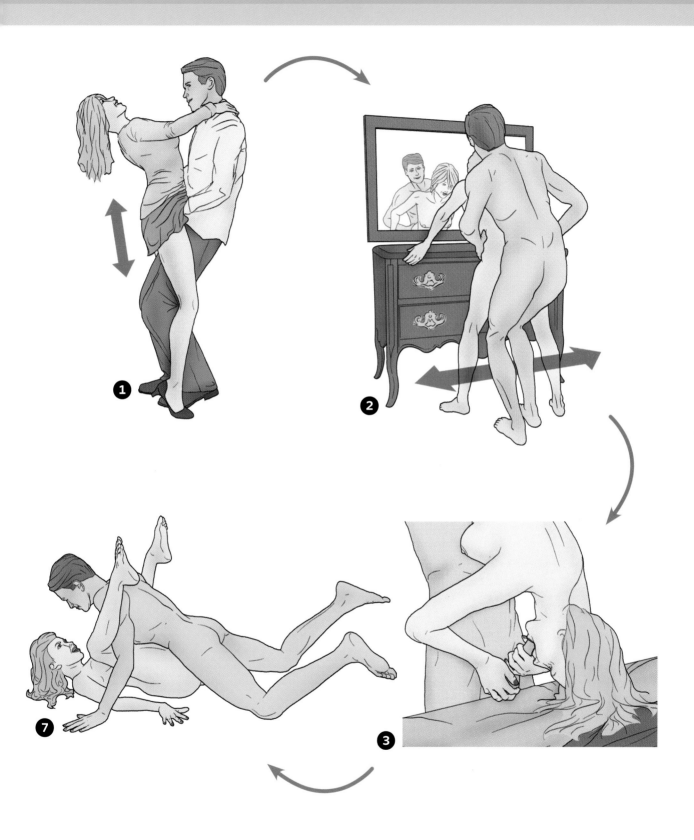

Resources

DVDS

Bend Over Boyfriend, Fatale Film, 1998.
A classic on how a woman can penetrate her male lover in specific detail.

BOOKS

Allison, Sadie. *Ride 'Em Cowgirl! Sex Position Secrets For Better Bucking*. San Francisco, CA, Tickle Kitty Press, 2007.
A sex-positive positions book, written in a light, humorous style.

Borg, Sonia. *Oral Sex He Will Never Forget*. Beverly, MA: Quiver Books, 2009.
This is the first book of the Never Forget series, which quickly became a bestseller. Hot scenarios to set the mood, tips from the Sexpert, and step-by-step moves make this a must read and the best he has ever had.

Borg, Sonia. *Oral Sex She Will Never Forget*. Beverly, MA: Quiver Books, 2010
The accompaniment to Oral Sex He Will Never Forget, which allows you to tell him what you like, without actually telling him. The scenarios teach him to set the mood and master foreplay, provides tips from the Sexpert, and step-by-step moves that will turn him into the best lover you have ever had. You have to train him, girl.

Corn, Laura. 101 *Sexy Dares*. New York City: Simon Spotlight Entertainment, 2008.
There are fifty dares for men and fifty dares for women. Each will give you inspiration to read and guaranteed fun if you dare to execute. The perforated pages add to the sense of excitement and adventure. A great buy.

Drake, Kypris Aster. *Journey to Sexual Wholeness: The Six Gateways to Sacred Sexuality*. San Diego, CA: Yabyummy Press, 2008.
Kypris candidly shares her own journey of enlightenment through sex and relationships. A wonderful book for anyone looking for something more in sexual experiences.

Kerner, Ian. *She Comes First: The Thinking Man's Guide to Pleasuring a Woman*. New York City. Harper Paperbacks, 2010.
A classic book that offers some very important fundamentals of pleasuring a woman, which are often overlooked, and more.

Lynn, Regina. *Sexier Sex: Lessons from the Brave New Sexual Frontier*. Berkeley, CA: Seal Press, 2008.
Great ideas on how to make sex more a part of your life, including tips on esex, phone sex, and much more.

Normandy, Marsha and Joseph St. James. *The Handjob Handbook*. New York: Simon Spotlight Entertainment, 2008.
Become a hand job expert in minutes with this simple and easy to grasp manual that includes the classic moves.

PRODUCTS AND SERVICES

JT's Stockroom
www.stockroom.com
A nice selection of BDSM gear at a fair price.

Good Vibrations

www.goodvibrations.com

The people at Good Vibrations know sex toys. The site offers excellent and useful information on sex and sex toys. More than just a store, all the employees are trained educators.

Juntos Personal Lubrication

www.juntoslubricants.com

Juntos offers quality, top-of-the-line products at an affordable price. You can't go wrong. Try to find the humping ladybugs on the website.

The Happy Endings Company

www.HotSexCoaching.com

This site includes free downloadable videos, books, and other affordable options for receiving sex coaching on a range of issues.

Monique Feil Photography

www.moniquefeil.com

Monique Feil is an artistic genius. She captures beauty like no photographer I've ever met and she gives you an unforgettable experience. Leave the photo session knowing you are beautiful and be reminded each time you look at the pictures. A must for every woman.

WEBSITES

Carnal Nation

www.carnalnation.com

Their slogan, "Personal, Political, Perverted" pretty much sums it up. Carnal Nation offers a refreshing perspective on sex and humor for your day.

The Kinsey Institute

www.kinseyinstitute.org

The Kinsey website shares some classic research that is valuable in the understanding of human sexuality to this day.

Society for Human Sexuality

www.sexuality.org

The objective of the Society for Human Sexuality (SHS) is to share sex-positive information over the internet. The site contains information and interviews from leading researchers and sexologists on topics such as safer sex, erotic massage, erotic talk, flirting, the G-spot, swing communities, and poly lifestyles.

Herpes Virus Association

www.herpes.org.uk

Don't let herpes get in the way of great sex. Most herpes websites are sponsored by pharmaceutical companies selling you fear so you buy their products. This is the best website I have found on the topic.

About the Author

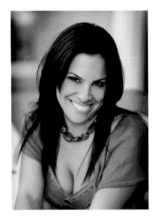

DR. SONIA BORG is a sex coach, clinical sexologist, best-selling author, speaker, and sex educator. She coaches clients to have their version of the best sex of their lives, both remotely and in person from her office.

Dr. Sonia earned her Ph. D. in human sexuality and masters in public health from The Institute for the Advanced Study of Human Sexuality in San Francisco and her masters degree in communication from San Francisco State University. Sonia is certified as a clinical sexologist by the American College of Sexologists and is a member of the American Association of Sexuality Educators Counselors and Therapists (AASECT).

Sonia has been featured on television and radio shows such as *Discovery Channel Canada*, *Playboy Radio*, *Good Morning San Diego*, and programs on KUSI in San Diego. She is the author of *Oral Sex He'll Never Forget* and *Oral Sex She'll Never Forget*.

Acknowledgments

A project of this magnitude would not be possible without the support from my faculty, colleagues, friends, and family.

I thank Ted McIlvenna for being my mentor and chair of my committee. I am truly honored. I appreciated his life wisdom, genuine caring, and delightful sense of humor.

I thank Marilyn Lawrence for serving on my committee. Her ability to listen, to be compassionate, and to offer guidance was appreciated.

I thank Harry Mohney for serving on my committee and providing feedback as a professional in the adult industry.

Interviews would not have been possible without the help of Ted McIlvenna, Harry Mohney, Peter Luster, club managers, and, of course, the dancers from coast to coast who responded to surveys and participated in interviews. The candor of the dancers was astounding and very much appreciated.

I got the best education in the humanities at IASHS and it is because of the caliber of faculty and fellow students. Thank you for being your best. It does make a difference. Thanks to the IASHS student group for your feedback and support. Although not on my committee, a special thanks to Howard Ruppel for caring and always suggesting ways to make my work better.

Thanks to Rand McIlvenna for capturing all my best angles on film and helping me feel comfortable in front of the camera.

A special thanks to Dr. Jerry Zientara for his keen eye and outstanding editing skills.

I am blessed with strong support system. Mom, Dad, Val, Rick, Patritzio, Joe, Adrianna, Tammy, Laura, Roe, and Deanna, thank you for being a part of my support system at an important time for me.